# CONTENTS

# PREFACE

Over recent years the need for health and social care professionals to work in different ways has become ever more evident as the context within which health and social care is delivered has changed. The momentum towards interprofessional working has increased significantly since the late 1990s, when the White Paper, *The New NHS, Modern – Dependable* (Department of Health, 1997) was published. This White Paper began a programme of modernization on a scale that had not been seen in the NHS since it was set up in 1948. In 2010, the coalition government announced major changes to the NHS which will herald a new era of opportunities and challenges for how health and social care services interact with each other. Importantly, the new ways of working have meant that interprofessional working is no longer optional, it is mandatory.

Changes affecting the workforce have already taken place, for example, the development of new and specialized roles, and these changes will continue to occur as the workforce develops and evolves. Traditional professional boundaries are being challenged, as health and social care professionals cross the boundaries to deliver patient-focused care using a team approach. To support these new ways of working, there have been radical changes to the education and training of health and social care professionals at both pre- and post-qualifying levels. The emphasis is on the interprofessional learning, with different professionals learning with, from and about each other in order to improve collaboration and thus enhance the quality of care provided. Significant organizational changes have also taken place to enable different agencies, notably, but not exclusively, the health services and social services, to work more effectively together.

Health and social care delivery is constantly in the spotlight and hardly a day goes by without the media making reference to a change that is proposed or has taken place. Sadly, all too often the media are reporting the tragic death of a vulnerable person that has occurred as a result of health and social care professionals not collaborating effectively.

There can be no doubt that interprofessional working can improve patient outcome, but change is uncomfortable and health and social care professionals are currently experiencing rapid and significant changes to both their working practices and to the environment within which they are working. This process of change will need to be carefully and sensitively managed if we are to achieve effective interprofessional working with an integrated patient-focused service.

Against this backdrop, this book is designed to provide you with the underpinning theoretical knowledge, understanding and skills to work effectively as a member of an interprofessional team. The book offers you practical advice and tips to help guide your practice to work and learn within an interprofessional context. There are two principal underpinning narrative threads:

- The developments in UK health and social care policy that have positioned interprofessional working at the centre of contemporary health and social care systems.

- The importance of ensuring that patients are the focus of care and that all health and social care professionals work as an integrated team to provide quality care in the best interests of the patient.

Each chapter explores a different aspect of interprofessional working. Chapter 1 uses an interprofessional practice-based scenario to introduce you to all the different aspects of interprofessional working. It also explores the semantic quagmire related to the term 'interprofessional'. In Chapter 2 we explore the context of interprofessional working and you will be introduced to all the relevant UK health and social care policies and legislation that are impacting on interprofessional developments in practice. Subsequent chapters deal with teams, team work and team dynamics; expertise and leadership; communicating with each other; learning within an interprofessional environment; and interprofessional learning within a practice environment. The final chapter of the book identifies the challenges to effective interprofessional working and offers practical suggestions for overcoming these barriers.

Within health and social care, various terms are used to refer to the person receiving care including patient, client and service user. For the sake of simplicity, in this book, the term patient will be used throughout. An Appendix at the back provides a table clearing mapping each chapter to the core NMC Standards and Essential Skills clusters. The book is also in line with the current vision and strategy of Jane Cummings, Chief Nursing Officer for England, that Nurses, Midwives and Care-Givers should have the following 'Six Cs' values to unite their professions: care; compassion; competence; communication; courage and commitment.

# ACKNOWLEDGEMENTS

I would like to take this opportunity to thank my friends and colleagues who helped and supported me while I wrote this book. I would particularly like to thank colleagues in both the School of Nursing and Midwifery and health and social care professionals from the practice setting who have provided practice scenarios, case studies and their thoughts on aspects of interprofessional working for inclusion in this book.

The publishers would like to thank Michelle Laing, Hilary Abbott-Bailey, Carolyn Crouchman and Richard Pitt for their insightful review comments on the manuscript.

# ABOUT THE AUTHOR

**Dr Jane Day** is currently Head of Division for Practice Learning and Midwifery, within the School of Nursing and Midwifery at University Campus, Suffolk. Her professional background is that of a therapeutic radiographer. Part of the responsibility within her current role is the management of the pre-registration Interprofessional Learning Programme provided for all pre-registration professional students at UCS, including nursing (adult, mental health and child), diagnostic radiography, therapeutic radiography, operating department practitioners, midwifery and social work, making interprofessional working one of her particular areas of expertise.

Series Editors for the *Nursing and Health Care Practice* Series:

**Dr Lynne Wigens**, Director of Nursing and Quality at The Ipswich Hospital NHS Trust. Visiting Senior Fellow University Campus Suffolk

**Dr Jane Day**, Head of Division, Practice Learning and Midwifery, School of Nursing and Midwifery, University Campus Suffolk

# WALK THROUGH TOUR

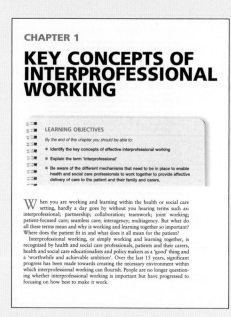

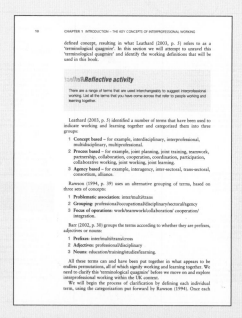

**Learning outcomes:** Listed at the beginning of each chapter, these emphasize the key topics that need to be understood before progressing to the next chapter.

**Key word definitions:** These are succinct definitions in the margin for important terms that are highlighted in the text.

**Reflective activity:** An opportunity to undertake structured reflection on the topics under discussion.

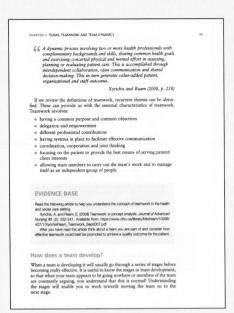

**Evidence base:** This provides well-founded evidence-based research about the topic for you to read.

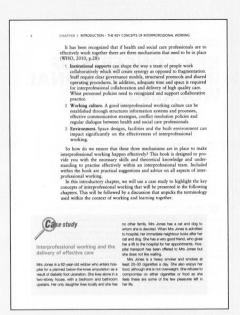

**Case study:** These are drawn from multi-professional settings to demonstrate scenarios and encourage you to think about how you practice and learn.

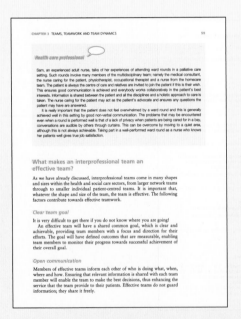

**Health care professional speaks:** A range of health care professionals talk about practical situations and caseload management issues (fictitious).

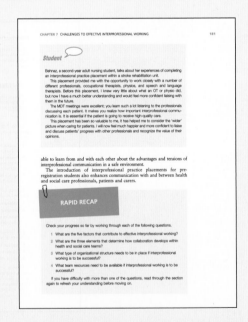

**Student speaks:** Students from a range of health care professions talk about their experiences of various situations (fictitious).

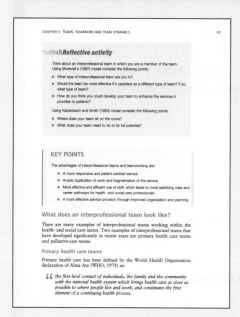

### Reflective activity

Think about an interprofessional team in which you are a member of the team. Using Øvretveit's (1997) model consider the following points.

* What type of interprofessional team are you in?
* Would the team be more effective if it operated as a different type of team? If so, what type of team?
* How do you think you could develop your team to enhance the services it provides to patients?

Using Katzenbach and Smith (1993) model consider the following points.

* Where does your team sit on the curve?
* What does your team need to do to its full potential?

### KEY POINTS

The advantages of interprofessional teams and teamworking are:

* A more responsive and patient-centred service
* Avoids duplication of work and fragmentation of the service
* More effective and efficient use of staff, which leads to more satisfying roles and career pathways for health- and social-care professionals
* A more effective service provision through improved organization and planning.

## What does an interprofessional team look like?

There are many examples of interprofessional teams working within the health- and social-care sector. Two examples of interprofessional teams that have developed significantly in recent years are primary health care teams and palliative-care teams.

### Primary health care teams

Primary health care has been defined by the World Health Organization declaration of Alma Ata (WHO, 1978) as:

> *the first level contact of individuals, the family and the community with the national health system which brings health care as close as possible to where people live and work, and constitutes the first element of a continuing health process.*

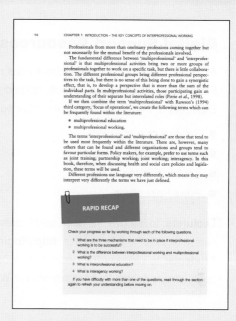

Professionals from more than one/many professions coming together but not necessarily for the mutual benefit of the professionals involved.

The fundamental difference between 'multiprofessional' and 'interprofessional' is that multiprofessional activities bring two or more groups of professionals together to work on a specific task, but there is little collaboration. The different professional groups bring different professional perspectives to the task, but there is no sense of this being done to gain a synergistic effect, that is, to develop a perspective that is more than the sum of the individual parts. In multiprofessional activities, those participating gain an understanding of their separate but interrelated roles (Pirrie *et al.*, 1998).

If we then combine the term 'multiprofessional' with Rawson's (1994) third category, 'focus of operations', we create the following terms which can be frequently found within the literature:

* multiprofessional education
* multiprofessional working.

The terms 'interprofessional' and 'multiprofessional' are those that tend to be used most frequently within the literature. There are, however, many others that can be found and different organizations and groups tend to favour particular forms. Policy makers, for example, prefer to use terms such as joint training; partnership working; joint working; interagency. In this book, therefore, when discussing health and social care policies and legislation, these terms will be used.

Different professions use language very differently, which means they may interpret very differently the terms we have just defined.

### RAPID RECAP

Check your progress so far by working through each of the following questions.

1 What are the three mechanisms that need to be in place if interprofessional working is to be successful?
2 What is the difference between interprofessional working and multiprofessional working?
3 What is interprofessional education?
4 What is interagency working?

If you have difficulty with more than one of the questions, read through the section again to refresh your understanding before moving on.

**Key points:** Summarize the main points in the preceding text.

**Rapid recap:** At the end of each chapter, these give the reader a chance to assess what they have learnt from reading the text. Answers are provided in the appendix.

## Digital Support Resources

All of our Higher Education textbooks are accompanied by a range of digital support resources. Each title's resources are carefully tailored to the specific needs of the particular book's readers. Examples of the kind of resources provided include:

- Self-test quiz questions
- Discussion Questions
- Critical Thinking Questions
- PowerPoint slides

**Lecturers:** to discover the dedicated lecturer digital support resources accompanying this textbook please register here for access: **http://login.cengage.com**.

**Students:** to discover the dedicated student digital support resources accompanying this text-book, please search for Interprofessional Working on: **www.cengagebrain.com**

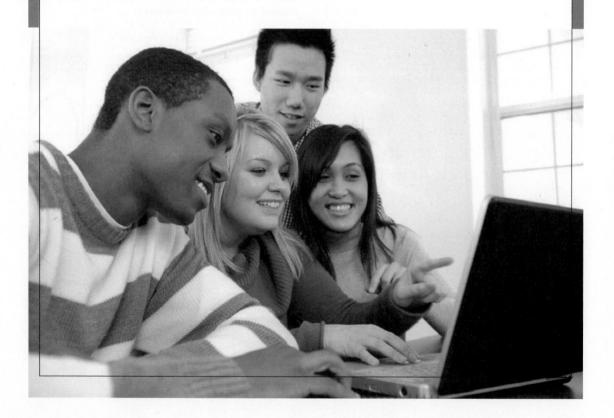

# CHAPTER 1

# KEY CONCEPTS OF INTERPROFESSIONAL WORKING

## LEARNING OBJECTIVES

*By the end of this chapter you should be able to:*

● Identify the key concepts of effective interprofessional working

● Explain the term 'interprofessional'

● Be aware of the different mechanisms that need to be in place to enable health and social care professionals to work together to provide effective delivery of care to the patient and their family and carers.

When you are working and learning within the health or social care setting, hardly a day goes by without you hearing terms such as: interprofessional; partnership; collaboration; teamwork; joint working; patient-focused care; seamless care; interagency; multiagency. But what do all these terms mean and why is working and learning together so important? Where does the patient fit in and what does it all mean for the patient?

Interprofessional working, or simply working and learning together, is recognized by health and social care professionals, patients and their carers, health and social care educationalists and policy makers as a 'good' thing and a 'worthwhile and achievable ambition'. Over the last 15 years, significant progress has been made towards creating the necessary environment within which interprofessional working can flourish. People are no longer questioning whether interprofessional working is important but have progressed to focusing on how best to make it work.

It has been recognized that if health and social care professionals are to effectively work together there are three mechanisms that need to be in place (WHO, 2010, p. 28):

1 **Institutional supports** can shape the way a team of people work collaboratively which will create synergy as opposed to fragmentation. Staff require clear governance models, structured protocols and shared operating procedures. In addition, adequate time and space is required for interprofessional collaboration and delivery of high quality care, whilst personnel policies need to recognize and support collaborative practice.

2 **Working culture** A good interprofessional working culture can be established through structured information systems and processes, effective communication strategies, conflict resolution policies and regular dialogue between health and social care professionals.

3 **Environment** Space designs, facilities and the built environment can impact significantly on the effectiveness of interprofessional working.

So how do we ensure that these three mechanisms are in place to make interprofessional working happen effectively? This book is designed to provide you with the necessary skills and theoretical knowledge and understanding to practise effectively within an interprofessional team. Included within the book are practical suggestions and advice on all aspects of interprofessional working.

In this introductory chapter, we will use a case study to highlight the key concepts of interprofessional working that will be presented in the following chapters. This will be followed by a discussion that unpicks the terminology used within the context of working and learning together.

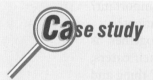
## Case study

### Interprofessional working and the delivery of effective care

Mrs Jones is a 62-year-old widow who enters hospital for a planned below-the-knee amputation as a result of diabetic foot ulceration. She lives alone in a two-storey house, with a bedroom and bathroom upstairs. Her only daughter lives locally and she has no other family. Mrs Jones has a cat and dog to whom she is devoted. When Mrs Jones is admitted to hospital, her immediate neighbour looks after her cat and dog. She has a very good friend, who gives her a lift to the hospital for her appointments. Hospital transport has been offered to Mrs Jones but she does not like waiting.

Mrs Jones is a heavy smoker and smokes at least 20–30 cigarettes a day. She also enjoys her food, although she is not overweight. She refuses to compromise on either cigarettes or food as she feels these are some of the few pleasures left in her life.

*Continued*

---

## BOX 1.1

There would appear to be an opportunity for health care professionals to promote a healthier lifestyle for Mrs Jones. Recent government policies and initiatives have focused on improving the health of the individual, and thus the population as a whole, with the emphasis being on preventative care. For example, a recommendation from the NHS Future Forum (Fields, 2012) is that every health and social care professional whatever his or her specialty should 'make every contact count'. This means every contact with a patient should be used as an opportunity to maintain or improve the patient's mental and physical health and well-being. As Mrs Jones smokes heavily all those professionals caring for her have a responsibility to advise her to stop smoking and offer her the necessary support should she wish to stop. Smoking cessation is a key part of the government's agenda for improving the public's health. The following government documents give a central place to smoking cessation services: the *NHS Smoking Cessation Services* (Department of Health, 2001); the *Choosing Health: Making Healthier Choices Easier* (Department of Health, 2004), the *Excellence in Tobacco Control: 10 High Impact Changes to Achieve Tobacco Control* (Department of Health, 2008) and the *Healthy Lives, Healthy People: our strategy for public health in England* (Department of Health, 2010). In Chapter 2 we will explore the health and social care policies and legislation which have encouraged interprofessional working and patient-centred care.

---

Mrs Jones has had Type 2 diabetes mellitus for 25 years, which is tablet controlled. However, her management of her diabetes is poor, which has resulted in her having had a stroke several years ago. The stroke affected her speech and impaired her mobility. Mrs Jones' mobility was already limited due to the ulceration of her foot. She uses a Zimmer frame to help her mobility. Her neighbour does her shopping for her, as Mrs Jones rarely leaves her house.

---

## BOX 1.2

Mrs Jones does not manage her diabetes very well. She could take advantage of, and may benefit from, attending a DESMOND (Diabetes Education and Self-Management for Ongoing and Newly Diagnosed) programme. This is a structured patient education programme for people with Type 2 diabetes and meets the criteria set down by NICE (2003) for suitable education programmes.

To support the development of structured education for people with diabetes, an interprofessional Diabetes UK Patient Education Working Group was set up in 2004. This group worked with the Department of Health and published the document, *Structured Patient Education in Diabetes* (Department of Health, 2005). The DESMOND education programme was one of the national programmes that resulted from this publication. This is another example of how health and social care policies have encouraged interprofessional working and patient-centred care.

## Continued

Mrs Jones has required previous hospital admissions for diabetic foot ulceration. These have been over a long period of time, which has resulted in Mrs Jones forming a dislike of all medical, nursing and physiotherapy staff. Mrs Jones is a very independent lady and her admissions to hospital have made her realize that, due to her condition, she is gradually losing her independence. She believes that she has been given contradictory information in the past by those health professionals caring for her and is, therefore, cynical about what they are telling her.

However, there are a few members of the interprofessional team that Mrs Jones does bond well with and she will communicate with these members of staff. These health care professionals are the diabetes nurse specialist, Susan, and one of her consultants, Dr Melson. Mrs Jones likes these two because they are straight talking and the language they use is easy to understand.

---

## BOX 1.3

Mrs Jones has indicated that she finds it difficult to understand all of the information being communicated to her by the health care professionals caring for her. Effective communication between health and social care professional and patient is considered essential for effective interprofessional working and the consequent delivery of quality health and social care to patients.

Professional language and jargon are often cited as a barrier to effective communication and therefore to interprofessional working. In Chapter 7, we will identify the challenges to effective interprofessional working and look at the impact that such barriers have on providing effective health and social care delivery.

---

Mrs Jones presents to the diabetic centre with an extensive ulcer in the region of her ankle, which has been non-healing for a number of months. The topical treatments that have been prescribed are not working. She is reviewed at the foot clinic, within the diabetes centre, and is seen jointly by her consultant, Susan (the diabetes nurse specialist) and a podiatrist (the diabetes team). Following the consultation, the diabetes team decide to offer Mrs Jones an angiogram/ angioplasty. As Mrs Jones trusts Susan, it is Susan who discusses the preferred treatment option with her. At first, Mrs Jones refuses to be admitted to hospital because it is close to Christmas. Eventually, she agrees to be admitted to hospital after Christmas.

*Continued*

## BOX 1.4

The diabetic team are all experts in their field. The consultant, diabetes nurse specialist and the podiatrist all contribute different but complementary knowledge, skills and expertise to the care of Mrs Jones. Each member of the team is aware of the roles and responsibilities of the others. In this case study, Susan, the diabetic nurse specialist, demonstrates some of the key characteristics of an expert: she is knowledgeable; she excels in her own domain; she values the participation of the consultant, podiatrist and district nurse in the decision-making process; and she is patient-centred in her approach.

It appears from the above that the diabetic team work well together and that, depending on the circumstance, different team members can take the lead. There appears to be a horizontal team structure as opposed to the traditional hierarchical team structure. In Chapter 4, Leadership and Expertise, we will discuss effective leadership; consider the complex nature of expertise and look at how expertise influences the leadership within an interprofessional team.

While Mrs Jones is waiting to be admitted, the district nurse continues to visit her on a daily basis, to clean and dress her ulcer. Mrs Jones has a 'communication book', which she takes with her to the diabetic centre. This book helps Susan to communicate with the district nurse who is caring for Mrs Jones on a daily basis.

## BOX 1.5

Mrs Jones' care is being shared between primary and secondary care teams. The majority of her care is provided within secondary (specialist) care, liaising with primary care. As we can see from this case study, the professionals in her primary care team include her GP; pharmacist; and district nurse. The professionals in her secondary care team include her consultant (with specialist training in diabetes), a podiatrist and a diabetes nurse specialist. The 'communication book' is one method of communication used by the primary and secondary care teams. Mrs Jones keeps the book, and she takes it to all her appointments at the diabetic clinic. The diabetes nurse specialist can write down suggestions on how to treat Mrs Jones' diabetic ulcer. The district nurse is then able to implement the suggestions made by the diabetes nurse specialist and can write in the book whether they worked or not. This is one method of communication and can enhance the effectiveness of teamwork. The district nurse and the diabetic nurse specialist will also communicate verbally, using the telephone. In Chapter 3 we will consider the different types of team, identify what helps and hinders effective teamwork and discuss the benefits of working in a team.

## *Continued*

Mrs Jones is admitted to hospital after Christmas and attends the radiology department for her angiogram. Susan is in attendance to provide moral support for Mrs Jones. During this investigation, Mrs Jones is uncommunicative with the staff in the radiology department, who have to rely on Susan for information. Susan believes that Mrs Jones is not communicating because she is scared about undergoing the investigation and is also afraid of the outcome of the angiogram.

Unfortunately, the result from the angiogram is not good. The diabetes team meet to discuss the preferred management option for Mrs Jones following the results. Mrs Jones is informed of the decision during a ward round. In attendance are her consultant, senior house officers, a nurse from the ward and Susan. The consultant explains to Mrs Jones that she will need to have a below-the-knee amputation. Mrs Jones does not ask any questions of any of the health care professionals in attendance. After the consultant has left, Susan explains the procedure to Mrs Jones, on a one-to-one basis. Mrs Jones communicates with Susan in a very matter-of-fact manner but it is obviously difficult for her to come to terms with losing part of her leg.

Following the operation, Mrs Jones' amputation heals well and there are no complications. Susan visits her on the ward on a daily basis to provide emotional support and discusses with Mrs Jones the practicalities of going home and living alone in her two-storey home.

The physiotherapist also visits Mrs Jones on a daily basis. Mrs Jones finds it difficult to get on with her physiotherapist, David, as she thinks that he does not understand how much her stroke is affecting her ability to mobilize.

The ward staff inform Susan, during one of her visits to the ward, that Mrs Jones has been abrupt and uncooperative. Mrs Jones believes that the ward staff have little insight into her situation. At this point Mrs Jones becomes very tearful, which improves the situation as it makes the ward staff realize that much of her perceived abruptness is purely a defence mechanism and it also allows Mrs Jones to see how supportive the ward staff are. Trips away from the ward with Susan appear to ease the tension. Going to the café provides the opportunity for Susan to chat with Mrs Jones in a relaxed environment. It is clear to Susan that Mrs Jones is very anxious to go home.

## BOX 1.6

As we have seen in this case study, Mrs Jones' previous experiences of attending hospital have not been positive and this has resulted in her finding it difficult to communicate with the health and social care professionals caring for her. Despite this, it is clear that all the professionals involved in her care communicate with her and try to involve her in the planning of her care and treatment. Susan, her diabetic nurse specialist, is a key health professional in Mrs Jones' care and, as we have seen, it is often Susan who communicates with the other health and social care professionals on her behalf. It is clear from the case study that the health and social care professionals involved in Mrs Jones' care and treatment liaise effectively with each other and that her pathway through the health and social care system is smooth and efficient.

In Chapter 5 we will explore the methods of communication which enhance effective interprofessional working, discuss the fundamental communication skills needed to facilitate effective relationships with service users and health care professionals and discuss the barriers to effective communication.

## *Continued*

Six weeks after her operation, a home assessment is arranged for Mrs Jones by an occupational therapist. Mrs Jones and the occupational therapist visit her home together and assess what adaptations need to be in place before she can be discharged home permanently. The adaptations required are minimal: her bed needs to be brought downstairs and a commode is necessary. However, leading up to Mrs Jones' front door is a very high step, which means that once in the house she cannot get out again. Mrs Jones is adamant that she wants to go home. It is agreed that she can be discharged provided that this is not a long-term solution and that more suitable accommodation is found very quickly.

Before Mrs Jones is discharged, she meets with a member of social services to start the process of finding alternative accommodation. Mrs Jones is discharged two weeks later and moves into a bungalow not long after going home.

## BOX 1.7

This case ends on a positive note, with Mrs Jones leaving hospital happy and with everything in place for her independent living. Her final contact with health care professionals is a positive one, which should mean that she will not be reluctant to come back into hospital should she need to.

An effective interprofessional team is evident in this case study and an integrated care package individualized for Mrs Jones has been provided. This case study demonstrates what can be achieved if health and social care professionals are working collaboratively with a patient-centred approach. In Chapter 6 we will consider the importance of interprofessional learning and look at ways in which a learning environment where effective interprofessional learning can take place can be created.

With reference to the case study:

● Draw a diagram to show the health and social care professionals who came into contact with Mrs Jones before she was admitted to hospital, while she was in hospital and after she was discharged.

● Consider how important the role of the diabetes nurse specialist was in providing care and support for Mrs Jones.

● How could the communication between Mrs Jones and the professionals caring for her have been enhanced?

● What further support could have been provided for Mrs Jones either before, during or after her stay in hospital?

## WHAT DOES THE TERM 'INTERPROFESSIONAL' MEAN?

At first this might seem like a straightforward question that would have a very straightforward unequivocal answer. However, this is not the case, with the literature revealing that the term 'interprofessional' is not a clearly defined concept, resulting in what Leathard (2003, p. 5) refers to as a 'terminological quagmire'. In this section we will attempt to unravel this 'terminological quagmire' and identify the working definitions that will be used in this book.

### *Reflective activity*

There are a range of terms that are used interchangeably to suggest interprofessional working. List all the terms that you have come across that refer to people working and learning together.

Leathard (2003, p. 5) identified a number of terms that have been used to indicate working and learning together and categorized them into three groups:

1 **Concept based** – for example, interdisciplinary, interprofessional, multidisciplinary, multiprofessional.
2 **Process based** – for example, joint planning, joint training, teamwork, partnership, collaboration, cooperation, coordination, participation, collaborative working, joint working, joint learning.
3 **Agency based** – for example, interagency, inter-sectoral, trans-sectoral, consortium, alliance.

Rawson (1994, p. 39) uses an alternative grouping of terms, based on three sets of concepts:

1 **Problematic association** – inter/multi/trans
2 **Grouping** – professional/occupational/disciplinary/sectoral/agency
3 **Focus of operations** – work/teamwork/collaboration/ cooperation/ integration.

Barr (2002, p. 30) groups the terms according to whether they are prefixes, adjectives or nouns:

1 **Prefixes** – inter/multi/trans/cross
2 **Adjectives** – professional/disciplinary
3 **Nouns** – education/training/studies/learning.

All these terms can and have been put together in what appears to be endless permutations, all of which signify working and learning together. We need to clarify this 'terminological quagmire' before we move on and explore interprofessional working within the UK context.

We will begin the process of clarification by defining each individual term, using the categorization put forward by Rawson (1994). Once each individual term has been defined, we will then combine terms and explore what the terms mean when related to learning and working together. This will provide a shared understanding of these terms that will help you understand the context within which this book refers to interprofessional working.

The first category we will consider is 'problem association':

- **Inter** – 'between, among; mutually; reciprocally' (*Oxford Dictionaries*, 2012).

  'denotes relationships both between and among the elements and further implies some notion of reciprocal operations' (Rawson, 1994, p. 40).

- **Multi** – 'more than one, many' (*Oxford Dictionaries*, 2012).

  'implies many and some form of composition but ... does not immediately suggest any give and take [within the group]' (Rawson, 1994, p. 40).

- **Trans** – 'across, beyond; through' (*Oxford Dictionaries*, 2012).

  'signifies relationships across or beyond but does not carry any indication of mutuality' (Rawson, 1994, p. 40).

Next we will consider the terms within the category 'grouping':

- **Professional** – 'relating to or belonging to a profession' (*Oxford Dictionaries*, 2012).

  Being a professional person is associated with particular distinctive features, which include:

  - membership of a restricted and regulated professional association, for example, Nursing and Midwifery Council (NMC), Health Care Professions Council (HCPC), General Medical Council (GMC).
  - having a great deal of autonomy
  - mastery of a specific body of knowledge, skills and expertise
  - an extensive period of education and training prior to practising
  - a philosophy of public service and altruism.

- **Occupational** – This is a broader term than 'professional', which leaves out the strong identity denoted by the term 'professional'.

- **Disciplinary** – The noun 'discipline' is defined as 'a branch of knowledge, especially one studied in higher education' (*Oxford Dictionaries*, 2012).

  The term 'disciplinary' suggests a narrower term than professional

- **Sectoral** – The noun 'sector' refers to 'an area or portion that is distinct from others, a distinct part of an economy, society or sphere of activity such as education' (*Oxford Dictionaries*, 2012).

  'Sectoral' refers to an organizational feature rather than a group of people

- **Agency** – 'a business or organization providing a particular service on behalf of another business, person or group' (*Oxford Dictionaries*, 2012).
- 'Agency', like 'sectoral', is referring to an organizational feature.
  It is a narrower term than 'sectoral', and its definition implies that there may be a number of agencies within a sector.

Finally we will consider the third of Rawson's (1994) categories, focus of operations

- **Collaboration** – 'the action of working with someone to produce something' (*Oxford Dictionaries*, 2012)
  'Collaboration' describes working together to achieve something that neither agency could achieve alone (Biggs, 1997, p. 188), whilst also pursuing their own organizational goals (Percy-Smith, 2005 cited in Atkinson *et al.*, 2007).
- **Cooperation** – 'the action or process of working together to the same end' (*Oxford Dictionaries*, 2012).
  'Cooperation' implies 'working together with positive connotations' (Biggs, 1997, p. 188)
- **Teamwork** – ' Teamwork is a dynamic process involving two or more health care professionals with complementary backgrounds and skills, sharing common health goals and exercising concerted physical and mental effort in assessing, planning, or evaluating patient care' (Xyrichis and Ream, 2008).

Having defined the individual terms we will combine some of them in an attempt to determine the definition we will use in this book to embody working and learning together.

Firstly, we will consider 'interprofessional' which is, of course, in the title of this book. If we put the definitions of 'inter' and 'professional' together we would come up with a definition such as the following:

> *Persons belonging to a profession, relating between and among each other, for the mutual benefit of those involved.*

This definition implies that if the different professional groups relate with each other there will be a synergist effect and that more will be achieved by the different groups relating with each other than if they were not. It must also be remembered that within any one workplace, the interprofessional relations need to take into account that there will be different professional groups working within the same organization and that the same professional groups will be working across different organizations. This begins to build up a picture of the complexity we are dealing with when we start to explore interprofessional working and learning.

However, before accepting this definition there needs to be further clarification of the term 'professional'. As noted earlier, historically there were only three professions, with others classed as semi-professions. If you continue to use such a restrictive definition of a profession, this will mean certain key groups will be excluded, for example police, teachers, patients and their carers, voluntary workers, leisure staff. All of these groups are important in the context of the well-being of people and therefore you would wish the term used to denote working and learning together to be an inclusive term. I would suggest, therefore, that within this book we use a less literal definition of a profession, to enable all groups that are working and learning together to provide health and social care for patients to be included within the term.

Combining 'inter' and 'professional' has combined two out of three of Rawson's (1994) categories. If we combine 'interprofessional' with terms from Rawson's (1994) third category 'focus of operations' we create terms such as:

- interprofessional learning
- interprofessional education
- interprofessional collaboration
- interprofessional teamwork.

All of these terms can be found within the literature. To work out the meaning of each term, you simply take the definition of 'interprofessional' and add it to the definition of the term from the third category, that is, collaboration, teamwork, education and learning.

Probably one of the most frequently used and widely accepted definitions of interprofessional education is that proposed by the Centre for the Advancement of Interprofessional Education (CAIPE, 2002):

> *Occurs when two or more professions learn with, from and about each other to improve collaboration and the quality of care.*

The World Health Organization (WHO, 2010) has adapted the CAIPE definition:

> *Occurs when two or more professions learn about, from and with each other to enable effective collaboration and improve health outcomes.*

As you can see the WHO definition extends beyond the quality of care to improve the health outcomes of people and populations.

In this book, however, when referring to interprofessional education, we will be using the CAIPE (2002) definition.

The next term that is frequently used within the literature is 'multiprofessional'. If we put together the definitions of 'multi' and 'professional', we would come up with a definition such as the following:

- Professionals from more than one/many professions coming together but not necessarily for the mutual benefit of the professionals involved.

The fundamental difference between 'multiprofessional' and 'interprofessional' is that multiprofessional activities bring two or more groups of professionals together to work on a specific task, but there is little collaboration. The different professional groups bring different professional perspectives to the task, but there is no sense of this being done to gain a synergistic effect, that is, to develop a perspective that is more than the sum of the individual parts. In multiprofessional activities, those participating gain an understanding of their separate but interrelated roles (Pirrie *et al.*, 1998).

If we then combine the term 'multiprofessional' with Rawson's (1994) third category, 'focus of operations', we create the following terms which can be frequently found within the literature:

- multiprofessional education
- multiprofessional working.

The terms 'interprofessional' and 'multiprofessional' are those that tend to be used most frequently within the literature. There are, however, many others that can be found and different organizations and groups tend to favour particular forms. Policy makers, for example, prefer to use terms such as joint training; partnership working; joint working; interagency. In this book, therefore, when discussing health and social care policies and legislation, these terms will be used.

Different professions use language very differently, which means they may interpret very differently the terms we have just defined.

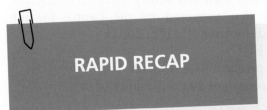

## RAPID RECAP

Check your progress so far by working through each of the following questions.

1  What are the three mechanisms that need to be in place if interprofessional working is to be successful?

2  What is the difference between interprofessional working and multiprofessional working?

3  What is interprofessional education?

4  What is interagency working?

If you have difficulty with more than one of the questions, read through the section again to refresh your understanding before moving on.

# REFERENCES

Atkinson, M., Jones, M. and Lamont, E. (2007) *working and its implications for practice: a review of the literature*. CfBT Education Trust.

Barr, H. (2002) *Interprofessional education: today, yesterday and tomorrow*. London: Learning and Teaching Support Network for Health Sciences and Practice.

Biggs, S. (1997) Interprofessional collaboration: problems and prospects' In Øvretveit, J., Mathias, P. and Thomson, T. (eds.). *Interprofessional working for health and social care*. London: Macmillan, pp. 186–200.

CAIPE (2002) Defining IPE available from: www.caipe.org.uk accessed May 2012.

Department of Health (2001) *NHS smoking cessation services. Service and monitoring guidance 2001/02*. London: HMSO.

Department of Health (2004) *Choosing health: making healthier choices easier*. London: HMSO.

Department of Health (2005) *Structured patient education in diabetes*. London: HMSO.

Department of Health (2008) *Excellence in tobacco control: 10 high impact changes to achieve tobacco control*. London: Central Office of Information.

Department of Health (2010) *Healthy lives, healthy people: our strategy for public health in England*. London: HMSO.

Fields, S. (2012) *NHS future forum. Summary report – second phase*. Available from www.dh.gov.uk/nhs-futureforum. Accessed July 2012.

Leathard, A. (2003) *Interprofessional collaboration: from policy to practice in health and social care*. London: Routledge.

NICE (2003) *Guidance on the use of patient education modules for diabetes*. London: NICE.

Oxford Dictionaries [online] (2012) Available at http://oxforddictionaries.com.

Pirrie, A., Wilson, V., Elsegood, J., Hall, J., Hamilton, S., Harden, R., Lee, D., and Stead, J. (1998) *Evaluating Multidisciplinary Education in Health Care*. Edinburgh, SCRE.

Rawson, D. (1994) Models of interprofessional work: likely theories and possibilities. In *Going interprofessional: working together for health and welfare* (ed. Leathard, A.). London: Routledge, pp. 38–63.

World Health Organization (2010) *Framework for action on interprofessional education and collaborative practice*. Switzerland: Health Professions Networks Nursing & Midwifery Office. Available from: http://www.who.int/hrh/resources/framework_action/en/index.html

Xyrichis, A. and Ream, E. (2008) Teamwork: a concept analysis. *Journal of Advanced Nursing* **61** (2): 232–241.

# CHAPTER 2
# INTERPROFESSIONAL WORKING CONTEXT

## LEARNING OBJECTIVES

*By the end of this chapter you should be able to:*

- Identify the relevant UK health and social care policies and legislation that are impacting on interprofessional developments in practice

- Understand the importance of participating effectively in interprofessional and multi-agency approaches to the delivery of health and social care

- Be aware of the historical circumstances that initiated the recent interprofessional developments.

## HISTORY OF INTERPROFESSIONAL DEVELOPMENTS

In this section we will trace the development of interprofessional working from when the National Health Service was first set up in 1948 through to the present day. Parallel to this we will consider the increase in service user involvement in developing health and social care services. In the UK over the past eighty years there has been a plethora of health and social care policies and legislation published which has helped to shape interprofessional working in partnership with the patients and their carers (Tope and Thomas, 2007). For simplicity's sake, therefore, only the key health and social care policies and legislation will be highlighted and discussed.

The value of collaboration between health, social care and employment was recognized in The Beveridge Report in 1942 which laid the foundation for the modern welfare state in the UK. Despite this report, however, the National Health Act 1946 and the National Assistance Act 1948 created a system whereby health and social care were separated rather than being brought together, a situation which remained until the end of the 1970s (Crawford, 2012). Through the 1960s,

1970s and the 1980s there was a flurry of activity related to interprofessional working by the government. It was not, however, until the mid 1990s that this flurry of activity became a rush with almost every Department of Health publication calling for health and social care professionals to work collaboratively.

It is important to remember that for the development of collaboration and effective interprofessional working, not only do the health and social care professionals need to want to collaborate, but also the organizational structures need to be in place for this to be possible. Health and social care policies, therefore, do not only need to encourage professionals to work together but also need to put the appropriate organizational structures in place.

## Key UK health and social care reports, policies and legislation

### The Younghusband Report, 1959

This report focused on the importance of health care teams collaborating with social workers for the benefit of patients and their families. The report also stated that good teamwork would be facilitated if there was an administrative structure which enabled co-operation between different departments.

The Younghusband Report was published over 50 years ago and 50 years on we are still hearing calls for health and social care professionals to develop more effective collaborative working.

### The Seebohm Report, 1968

This report recommended that the differences between children's and adult services should be reduced by placing them all under amalgamated local authority services departments (Crawford, 2012). It also identified that closer working relationships between social services and general practitioners was desirable.

### The Alma Ata Declaration (World Health Organization, 1978)

The Alma Ata Declaration was defined following a World Health Organization conference on primary health care held in Alma Ata in the former USSR. The declaration called for a more holistic approach to primary care to be taken, with the establishment of community health centres and community health workers.

This declaration placed the patient and their family and carers at the centre of their care, encouraging them to fully participate in the discussions and decisions made about care and treatment, that is, a patient-focused care approach was being advocated.

### Working for Patients (Department of Health, 1989a)

This White Paper outlined the most significant cultural shift that the NHS had seen since its inception in 1948, with the introduction of the internal market.

The internal market gave 'purchasers' (health authorities and some GPs) budgets to buy health care from 'providers' (acute hospitals; organizations providing care for the mentally ill, the elderly, people with learning disabilities; and ambulance services). To become a 'provider', health organizations became NHS Trusts, independent organizations with their own managements, competing with each other. This White Paper began to make the organizational changes that were required to make interprofessional working possible.

## Caring for People: Community Care in the Next Decade and Beyond (Department of Health, 1989b)

This White Paper gave the lead responsibility for community care to local authorities but it recognized that there was an important interface with other key services, particularly those of the NHS. The White Paper, therefore, placed an emphasis on joint working in order for health and social care services to be jointly responsible for the provision of care in the community.

## The NHS and Community Care Act 1990

The NHS and Community Care Act 1990 made the legal changes necessary for the new arrangements set out in the White Papers, *Working for Patients* (Department of Health, 1989a) and *Caring for People: Community Care in the Next Decade and Beyond* (1989b).

## The New NHS, Modern – Dependable (Department of Health, 1997)

This White Paper signalled the biggest programme of change the NHS had seen since its inception in 1948. Following the election of a new government in 1997, Tony Blair declared that the publication of this White Paper was to be a turning point for the NHS and was the start of a process of modernization.

After 50 years of policies and legislation designed to encourage health and social care professionals to work with each other and across services and agencies, including the voluntary and private sector, this White Paper provided the necessary impetus for interprofessional working to become a reality.

The White Paper announced an end to the inequities and inefficiencies of the internal market, replacing it with a system of integrated care based on partnership and driven by performance.

To facilitate the development of integrated care, the White Paper reported that organizational barriers would be broken down and that patients would no longer be passed back and forth between different agencies with competing agendas. The claim was that cooperation would replace competition and that the NHS would forge new working relationships locally with education, employment, housing and social services.

This White Paper was essentially about putting patients at the heart of the NHS and moving the focus from a service that does things to and for its patients to one that works with patients.

If we review this White Paper, we can see that three main themes emerge:

1 partnership working
2 patient-centred care
3 organizational changes to make themes one and two possible.

Thus, in 1997, new ways of working and collaboration on a scale not previously seen within the NHS began to be introduced and until 2010 health and social care policies have set out the changes which need to be made within the NHS and social services in order to implement the vision laid out within this White Paper.

## *Modernizing Social Services* (Department of Health, 1998a)

In this White Paper the importance of social services working in partnership with statutory agencies, voluntary organizations and independent providers to create a system of integrated care which put users and their carers at the centre of service provision was discussed. The White Paper also outlined legislative changes to make joint working easier.

This White Paper clearly demonstrates the three main themes, that is, partnership, patient-centred care and organizational change, that were identified in the White Paper, *The New NHS, Modern – Dependable* (Department of Health, 1997) as being essential for the modernization of the NHS.

## *A First Class Service: Quality in the new NHS* (Department of Health, 1998b)

The National Service Frameworks (NSFs) were one of the developments that arose from this White Paper. There are currently nine NSFs which have been rolled out between 1999 and 2006. NSFs cover the following conditions: diabetes, coronary heart disease, long term conditions, chronic obstructive pulmonary disease and renal disease and the following key patient groups: children, young people and maternity, mental health and older people.

One strength of the NSFs is that they were developed in partnership with health professionals, patients, carers, health service managers, voluntary agencies and other experts. Partnership is a key theme within all the NSFs. For example, *National Service Framework for Older People* (Department of Health, 2001a) advocated a single assessment process. The need for each health and social care professional to undertake his or her own assessment of an older person was no longer required. This means that a single, tailored care package can be developed for the older person and be delivered by specialist networks of professionals working across primary, community and hospital settings. The *National Service Framework for Children, Young People and Maternity* (Department of Health, 2004a) aimed to ensure that the care the child and their parents and/or carers receive is better coordinated, so that they do not have to see too many professionals and repeat their story over and over again.

### The Health Act 1999 – Modern Partnerships for People (Department of Health, 1999a)

The Health Act 1999 provided new powers to enable health and local authority partners to work together more effectively. These new powers were referred to as flexibilities. The purpose of the flexibilities was to enable partners, for example health bodies (Primary Care Trusts, Strategic Health Authorities) and any health-related local authority services (social services, community and acute services, housing) to join together to design and deliver services around the needs of the patient rather than worrying about the boundaries of their organizations. These arrangements were designed to eliminate unnecessary gaps and duplications between services.

### Agenda for Change: Modernizing the NHS Pay System (Department of Health, 1999b)

Differences in payment, conditions of service and rewards have been cited as a barrier to interprofessional working. *Agenda for Change* was a radical change to the pay system for all staff directly employed by the NHS, with the exception of very senior managers and those covered by the Doctors' and Dentists' Pay Review Body. The new pay system was designed to overcome these barriers.

### Primary Care Trust (PCTs): Establishing Better Services (Department of Health, 1999c)

PCTs were established to provide a range of benefits to patients, the community and professionals including:

- Development of multidisciplinary education and training programme which support the continuing professional development of practice staff.
- Sharing of resources and skills among primary care and community professionals
- Better integrated services including the development of intermediate care
- Bringing decision making closer to patients and local communities.

In England 302 PCTs were established with his number being reduced to 152 in 2006 as part of the government's drive to create a patient-led NHS. The PCTs are scheduled to be abolished in 2013 with GP-led Commissioning Consortia taking on most of the commissioning responsibility (Department of Health, 2010a).

### The NHS Plan: A plan for investment, a plan for reform (Department of Health, 2000)

It was not until *The NHS Plan* was published in 2000 that the plans to transform the NHS as described in the White Paper, *The New NHS, Modern – Dependable* (Department of Health, 1997) came into focus. This White Paper described a ten-year plan that was designed to tackle the systemic problems of the NHS which dated from when it was formed in 1948. These systemic problems included most notably old-fashioned demarcations between staff and barriers between services.

Reforms included within *The NHS Plan* designed to enhance interprofessional working included:

- Creation of Care Trusts to provide better-integrated health and social care. Care Trusts, an NHS body, are designed to bring the NHS responsibilities and local authority health responsibilities together under a single management structure. This structural change in health and social care provision was designed to increase continuity of care and simplify administration. Care Trusts were introduced in 2002 and at present there are 11 Care Trusts in England.
- Nurses and other staff are to have a greater opportunity to extend their roles. This reform was designed to develop a flexible workforce, where multiple professionals are able to take on tasks traditionally seen as the domain of one profession. Since the publication of *The NHS Plan*, there have been a host of new roles created, including assistant practitioners; advanced practitioners; non-medical consultants, in, for example, radiography, nursing, midwifery and health visiting; non-medical prescribing for nurses and allied health professionals; community matrons and modern matrons.

### The Health and Social Care Act 2001 (Department of Health, 2001b)

This Act was the legislation that allowed the reforms outlined in *The NHS Plan* (Department of Health, 2000) to be taken forward. The Act covered a range of measures related to primary care, long-term care of the elderly, patient advocacy, nurse prescribing and the creation of Care Trusts.

### The NHS Improvement Plan: Putting People at the Heart of Public Services (Department of Health, 2004b)

In this publication, the Department of Health once again pledged their commitment to greater flexibility and growth in the way services are provided, which will be matched by increases in NHS staff and new ways of working to meet patients' needs.

### Our Health, Our Say, Our Care: A New Direction for Community Services (Department of Health, 2006)

This White Paper built on two previous White Papers, *Saving Lives Our Healthier Nation* (1999e) and *Choosing Health* (2004b). It was designed to reform and improve community services, to create health and social care services that genuinely focus on prevention and promoting health and well-being; that deliver care in more local settings; that promote the health of all, not just a privileged few; and that deliver services that are flexible, integrated and responsive to peoples' needs and wishes.

### High Quality Care for All: NHS Next Stage Review (Department of Health, 2008a)

In this document a ten-year vision for a world class NHS that is fair, personally effective and safe was outlined. The principles and values of this White Paper include:

- NHS services must reflect the needs and preferences of patients, families and their carers.
- The NHS works across organizational boundaries and in partnership with other organizations in the interest of patients, local communities and the wider population.

### High Quality Workforce: NHS Next Stage Review (Department of Health, 2008b)

This White Paper defines how the quality of care provided for patients will be enhanced through the NHS, Higher Education sector and industry working together to improve the quality of education and training offered in the NHS. This document addresses needs across the whole of the NHS workforce and links to social care, recognizing that teams work increasingly with others, particularly social care workers.

### Health and Social Care Act, 2008 (Department of Health, 2008c)

This Act contained significant measures to modernize and integrate health and social care. This included the creation of the Care Quality Commission (CQC), a single, independent, integrated regulator for health and social care in England. The CQC replaced previous monitoring and inspection bodies. At the heart of the CQC work is the desire for the voices of the people who use health and social care to be heard.

### Equity and Excellence: Liberating the NHS (Department of Health, 2010a)

Following the election of the coalition government in the UK in 2010 the most sweeping changes in the history of the NHS were announced in this White Paper. The emphasis was still very much focused on successful integration of health and social care. Significant changes to the structure of the NHS have been announced to facilitate this integration including: the creation of general practitioner consortia, a national commissioning board and local health and being boards.

## *A Vision for Adult Social Care: Capable Communities and Active Citizens* (Department of Health, 2010b)

This White Paper sets out a vision for adult social care which is built on seven principles: prevention, personalization, partnership, plurality, protection, productivity and people (Department of Health, 2010 p. 8). This document emphases the three main themes that emerged from *The New NHS: Modern – Dependable* (1997):

1 Partnership working
2 Patient-centred care
3 Organizational changes to make themes one and two possible.

## *The Health and Social Care Act 2012* (Department of Health, 2012)

This Act puts clinicians at the centre of commissioning, frees up providers to innovate, empowers patients and gives a new focus to public health.

As can be seen from this historical overview, from 1942 when the Beveridge Report was published, the importance of partnerships between NHS organizations, social services and the voluntary and private sectors has been recognized. However, up until 1997, when the White Paper, *The New NHS, Modern – Dependable* (Department of Health, 1997) was published the organizational structures and the ways in which the professions were working were not conducive to interprofessional working. Since 1997 this has been changing and new organizational structures and new ways of working have been evolving. In 2010, the coalition government announced major changes to the NHS which will herald a new era of opportunities and challenges for how health and social care services interact with each other. Importantly, the new ways of working have meant that interprofessional working is no longer optional, it is mandatory.

As stated at the beginning of this historical overview, only the key health and social care policies related to interprofessional working have been discussed in this section. This section has not included those health and social care policies related to specific services, for example children's services and mental health services. For these two services, there have been many health and social care policies and legislation that have shaped the partnership approach taken to the care provided for patients.

## THE 'DRIVERS' OF INTERPROFESSIONAL WORKING

Changes in professional practice do not occur in isolation, they are always located in a social, economic and political context. It is important to consider why we have interprofessional working and who benefits.

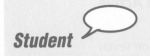

*Student*

Kelly, a student midwife talks of her experiences of interprofessional working and woman centre care. The Special Care Baby Unit (SCBU) has a multidisciplinary team (MDT) meeting every morning. SCBU is divided into two bays, first bay is for intensive care and high dependency and second is a low dependency bay. The team start in the high dependency bay and will ask all visitors and parents to leave, so that the doors can be closed to maintain confidentiality. In turn each baby's parents will be asked to return when it is time for their baby to be discussed. The doctor will commence an outline of the baby's medical condition and state what has occurred over the past day, the consultant for that baby will then do some general observations of that baby. They will also get advice from the dietician and engage with the nursing staff, sister and parents to make a plan for the baby for that day. Once the baby has been seen and discussed and a plan made the consultant will make sure the parents are happy and then the next baby will be discussed and that baby's parents invited in.

These ward rounds appear to work very well as the patient is in front of them, rather than discussing from another room. Also because there is a huge wealth of knowledge available from the MDT who can advise and help make a plan for the baby's care. Another hurdle that has been overcome with ward rounds is the issue of confidentiality, as only the MDT and nursing staff are permitted in the bay whilst the ward round is in progression, with each individual baby's parents invited into the bay to be a part of this and asked to leave once finished.

In the past, while different professionals have worked alongside one another, caring for an individual patient, they were not seen as part of a team, and teamwork was, therefore, not evident.

Over recent years the requirement for health and social care professionals to work interprofessionally has become ever more evident, as the context within which health and social care is delivered has changed. The drivers for interprofessional working include:

1  the voice of the patient
2  policies and initiatives
3  poor collaborative practice
4  professional developments
5  technological developments.

## 1. The voice of the patient

As we have seen earlier in this chapter successive White Papers have placed the patient at the centre of the NHS empowering patients to have a direct input into the care they receive. This has fundamentally changed the way in which health and social care practitioners practise and collaborative working is essential if the needs of the patients are to be met. In addition to the White Papers already discussed, other initiatives have provided a greater voice for the patient to influence the care they receive:

## Local Involvement Networks (LINks) set up in 2008 (Department of Health, 2007a)

These are made up of individuals and community groups, such as charities, faith groups, and residents' associations and youth councils, who work together to improve local health and social care services.

LINks will be abolished in April 2013 (Department of Health, 2010a) and be replaced by Local Healthwatch. Local Healthwatch will take on the work of LINks and will also:

- Represent the views of people who use services, carers an the public on Health and Wellbeing boards set up by local authorities
- Provide a complaint advocacy service
- Report concerns about quality of health care to Health Watch England which can recommend that Care Quality Commission (CQC) take action.

*(www.cqc.org.uk)*

- Healthwatch England set up in 2012 (Department of Health, 2010a)
  Healthwatch England is an independent consumer champion created to gather and present the views of the public. It will play a role at both national and local levels and will make sure that the views of the public and people who use services are taken into account.

## Reflective activity

Reflect on stories in the national media concerning patient care and consider the following:

- The main concerns that have been expressed.
- Is there is any evidence to suggest that lack of interprofessional collaboration impacted on the quality of care provided for the patients
- Think about how interprofessional collaboration could be strengthened
- The action you would take to raise a concern about the quality of care you were observing.

- National Voices (www.nationalvoices.org.uk)
  National Voices is the coalition of health and social care charities in England. It works together to strengthen the voices of patients, service users, carers, their families and the voluntary organizations that work for them. National Voices seeks to narrow the gap between the rhetoric about patient centred care and reality and champions voice, choice and involvement; a seamless service; fairness and justice, safety and quality.

## EVIDENCE BASE

Go to the following website **http://healthandcare.dh.gov.uk/what-is-healthwatch/** and find out more about Healthwatch England

Find out more about Local Healthwatch by reading the following document:

Local Healthwatch: A strong voice for people – the policy explained. This document can be accessed at **http://healthandcare.dh.gov.uk/files/2012/03/Local-Healthwatch-policy.pdf**

## 2. Policies and initiatives

Over the last ten years, the Department of Health has published many White Papers which have set out proposals to encourage teamwork and interprofessional working both between and within health and social care provision.

The *National Service Frameworks* (Department of Health, 1998c) have increased interprofessional models of care in areas such as diabetes, stroke, obesity, end of life and dementia. Growing problems associated with domestic violence, anti-social behaviour, alcohol and substance dependency and homelessness have also increased the necessity to work collaboratively across health and social care, for example children and adolescent mental health services, youth offending teams, drug and alcohol action teams.

A focus on improving the health of the population as a whole, with the emphasis being on preventative care has also increased the necessity for interprofessional working. Initiatives such as Sure Start, Change4life, smoking cessation programmes and Chlamydia screening programmes have been implemented.

If these initiatives are to be successful in providing innovative approaches to health and social care in the community, it is crucial that there is effective collaboration between the NHS, local authorities, social services, the private and voluntary sector and industry.

These initiatives illustrate that the government continues to vehemently encourage and believe that effective interprofessional working will result in the effective delivery of patient-centred approaches to health and social care.

The previous section, 'Historical overview of interprofessional developments', provides more detail on the health and social care policies and legislation that have shaped interprofessional working in the UK.

## 3. Poor collaborative practice

The tragic deaths of young people as a result of abuse are all too frequently hitting the national headlines. In the UK, at least one child dies every week as a result of abuse. Many of these deaths never hit the national headlines, but they are no less tragic than those cases which do. Many other children suffer humiliating, dehumanizing and degrading experiences from people on whom they are totally dependent, their main carers.

One of the earliest reported deaths was that of Dennis O'Neill (Monckton Report, 1948, cited in Hopkins, 2007) who died at the hands of his foster father. This was almost 65 years ago and yet the tragic deaths have continued to occur, one of the most recent being Baby Peter who died in 2007 (Laming, 2009) who died at the hands of his mother, her boyfriend and a family lodger. Other tragic deaths include Maria Colwell, 1973; Jasmine Beckford, 1984; children undergoing heart surgery at Bristol Royal Infirmary, 1984–1995; Kimberley Carlie, 1986; Doreen Mason, 1987; Leanne White, 1992; Riki Neave, 1994; Chelsea Brown, 1999; Lauren Wright, 2000; Victoria Climbié, 2000; Ainlee Labonte, 2002; Tyrell Rowe, 2003; Kimberley Baker, 2005 and Tiffany Wright, 2007.

Following the death of Dennis O'Neill in 1945, a Home Office inquiry (The Monckton Report, 1945) identified a string of failures by the staff and agencies involved in the case. There was confusion between the two local authorities responsible for Dennis O'Neill's foster placement, conflicting reports by childcare staff on his wellbeing, staff shortages and miscommunications.

The key messages from this report were that there needed to be better collaboration across organizational boundaries and improved communication between professionals.

Almost 30 years after the report into the death of Dennis O'Neill, the report into the death of Maria Colwell (Department of Health and Social Security, 1974, p. 86) concluded that the 'greatest and most obvious' failure of the system was 'the lack of, or effectiveness of communication and liaison'. This report also highlighted that the social worker involved in this case had a lack of knowledge and that training was, therefore, an issue. As can be seen, sadly, the same issues, lack of collaboration between agencies and lack of communication between professionals, which were present in 1948, were still present in 1974.

Another 30 years on from the death of Maria Colwell, the report into the death of Victoria Climbié (Laming, 2003) depressingly concluded by raising the same major issues. The Report, which concluded with 108 recommendations, highlighted a lack of collaborative working between agencies, a lack of effective sharing of information, and generally poor communication and lack of training of medical staff and in particular general practitioners (GPs).

In 2007, seven years after the death of Victoria Climbié, Baby Peter died. Both children lived in the same London Borough of Haringey. The report by Laming (2009) into his death had among its recommendations:

- All Children's Trusts should have multi-agency training to create a shared language and understanding of local referral procedures. A named child protection lead in each setting should receive this training.
- Children's Trusts must ensure that all assessments include evidence from all the professionals involved, take account of case histories and include direct contact with the child.
- Every Children's Trust should ensure that partners consistently apply the Information Sharing Guidance.
- Children's Trusts must ensure police, community paediatric specialists and health visitors send representatives to act as partners to children's services departments.

As can be seen, each new inquiry into a child's death over the last 65 years has resulted in a new but recurring set of recommendations. Sadly, it is apparent that the same issues exist today:

- lack of collaboration between agencies
- lack of effective communication
- lack of adequate training.

Unfortunately, these deficits in interprofessional working are not specific to child protection. Reports into failures in mental health care, for example the death of Father Paul Bennett who was killed by Geraint Evans, paranoid schizophrenic (Health care Inspectorate Wales, 2009) and the death of a ten-day-old baby boy by his mother, Katy Norris who was suffering from severe post natal depression (Torbay Safeguarding Children Board, *Serious Case Review*, 2010) also reported lapses in collaboration, ineffective communication and inadequate training as impacting on the quality of care that these patients received.

In addition to the child abuse and mental health examples there are other high profile examples whereby deaths could have been prevented with better training, communication and monitoring systems. For example, the inquiry into the children undergoing heart surgery at Bristol Royal Infirmary (Secretary of State for Health, 2001) recommended that:

- Education in communication skills must be an essential part of the education of all health care professionals. Communication skills include the ability to engage with patients on an emotional level, to listen, to assess how much information a patient wants to know and to convey information with clarity and sympathy.
- Communication skills must include the ability to engage with and respect the views of fellow health care professionals.

In 2000 Harold Shipman, a GP in Hyde was convicted of the murder of 15 of his patients. There were five separate Shipman inquiries with reports published between 2002 and 2005. The First report published in 2002 noted that:

> *It is deeply disturbing that Shipman's killing of his patients did not arouse suspicion for so many years. The systems which should have safeguarded his patients against his misconduct, or at least detected misconduct when it occurred, failed to operate satisfactorily. The esteem in which Shipman was held ensured that very few relatives felt any real sense of disquiet about the circumstances of the victims' deaths. Those who did harbour private suspicions felt unable to report their concerns. It was not until March 1998 that any fellow professional felt sufficiently concerned to make a report to the coroner.*

*Smith (2001)*

The inquiry found systems failures, which enabled Shipman, despite having a drugs conviction, to stockpile controlled drugs, and bypass the normal coroner's investigations, which allowed his activities to go unchecked by other professionals over many years. This case clearly demonstrated that there were inadequacies in the regulation of medical practitioners at this time and that the systems in place that should provide the necessary checks and balances for the professionals involved were not sufficiently robust.

However, underpinning the difficulties just described are fundamental organizational and structural problems, which need to be addressed in order to facilitate interprofessional working. When the Welfare State was created in the 1940s, health and social services were separated administratively at both central and local levels. This has meant that ever since the inception of the Welfare State, health and social services have had to make continual attempts to ensure their coordination. Over the years, health and social care policies have sought to encourage the coordinated planning of health and social services. Recently, however, this has gained an increased momentum with the publication of *Equity and Excellence: Liberating the NHS* (Department of Health, 2010a) and *A Vision for Adult Social Care: Capable Communities and Active Citizens* (Department of Health, 2010b). The significance of these health and social care policies and legislation for interprofessional working is discussed above in 'Historical overview of interprofessional developments'.

## 4. Professional developments

Health and social care provision has become increasingly complex to ensure that the needs of the patient continue to be met. Consequent to this growth in complexity, there has been an expansion in the knowledge and skills of those health and care professionals delivering the care. This expansion of knowledge has led to increased specialization within the health and social care professions and new roles are being developed, for example clinical nurse specialists and consultant radiographers. As a result, teams with a greater skill-mix now deliver care to patients. If this team delivery approach is to be successful, effective interprofessional collaboration is essential.

The number of professionals available has also led to new specialist roles and subsequent new ways of working. For example, the current lack of availability of doctors means that if the traditional model of providing health and social care is maintained, future expectations for the delivery of quality care are unlikely to be met. It is, therefore, more likely that the availability of professionals will shape future patterns of service delivery. Delivery will be provided in such a way that it ensures that the skills of all team members are used, by allowing them to contribute to their full potential.

Professional developments have impacted, and will continue to impact, on the nature of the delivery of care. These developments will inevitably mean that the traditional professional boundaries will be challenged as professionals cross the boundaries to deliver care to patients, using a team approach.

## 5. Technological developments

Although technological developments are not the drivers for interprofessional teamwork, they do have the potential to significantly enhance and influence interprofessional health and social care delivery. The use of information technology, for example mobile telephones, e-mail facilities, electronic patient records and video conferencing, will have a major impact on the development of interprofessional collaboration in primary health care. As members of primary health care teams are not usually geographically close to one another, advances in information technology will mean that information can be transferred more easily between members of the health care team. This will provide better opportunities for consultation between primary health care professionals, reduce professional isolation and should ultimately result in enhanced patient care.

These technological developments have also significantly increased the information available to patients. No longer are patients basing their decisions only on information provided by local health and social care providers, they also have access to information across the world. To meet these changing needs and the expectations of patients, there is a requirement for more sophisticated approaches to the delivery of care involving effective teamwork, with health and social care professionals crossing boundaries and working interprofessionally.

Advances in telecommunications and information technology will inevitably have an important role to play in developing and sustaining interprofessional working.

## INITIATIVES TO ENCOURAGE INTERPROFESSIONAL WORKING

In this section, we will discuss two examples of specific initiatives from the health and social care sectors to explore the impact that health and social care policies and legislation have had on interprofessional working within the practice environment. The two initiatives selected are:

1 Sure Start
2 Stroke

## 1. Sure Start

Sure Start launched in 1998 was an initiative which originated from the government's *Cross Department Review of Provision for Young Children*

(HM Treasury, 1998). The aim of Sure Start was to tackle child poverty and social exclusion through integration and co-ordination of services in early education, childcare, and health, employment and family support for pre-school children and their families. The Department for Education and Employment (1999, p. 6) stated:

> " Providers of services and support will work together in new ways that cut across old professional and agency boundaries and focus more successfully on family and community needs

Sure Start is one initiative within a broad range of government policies designed to develop collaborative and integrated service provision to better meet the needs of children and young people (Edgley and Avis, 2007). These policies include The Children Act, 2004, *Every Child Matters* (Department for Education and Skills, 2004) and the *National Service Framework for Children, Young People and Maternity Services* (Department of Health, 2004a).

During 1999 to 2003, 524 Sure Start Local Programmes (SSLPs) were set up across England, providing services for families living within a specified postcode (Edgley and Avis, 2007). As SSLPs delivered services tailored to meet the needs of families living within their area prioritizes varied from programme to programme, but the work of all the SSLPs was targeted at:

- Improving learning
- Improving children's health
- Improving social and emotional development
- Strengthening families and communities
- Increasing childcare provision – added in 2005

*Sure Start Unit (2001)*

In 2004 Sure Start Children Centres (SSCCs) were established to contribute to achieving the outcomes of *Every Child Matters* (Department for Education and Skills, 2004). This was a national initiative aimed at all families with children under five, rather than the previous focus on 'deprived' communities. The majority of SSLPs became SSCCs and new SSCCs were created to meet the government's goal of having a Children Centre for every community. The current coalition government has indicated its commitment to SSCCs although it has proposed a move away from the 'universal' Children Centre model towards a targeting of services at the 'neediest' and most vulnerable children and families (Asthana, 2010 cited in Lloyd and Harrington, 2012).

Box 2.1 illustrates the vast range of services and activities that are delivered nationally by SSCCs.

## BOX 2.1

### Range of services provided by Sure Start Children Centres

- Parents and toddler groups
- Parenting course and support
- Dad's groups
- Employment and training for parents – links with Jobcentre Plus
- Help to stop smoking
- Groups for teenage parents
- Support for children with additional needs and their families
- Breast feeding peer support
- Outreach and home visiting support

- Speech and language development support
- In depth family support
- Advice on healthy eating
- High quality childcare and early learning provision
- Advice on money
- Antenatal sessions
- Toy library
- Sensory room
- Drop in child health clinics

References: National Audit Office, 2006; Malin and Morrow, 2007; Edgley and Avis, 2007

To enable the SSCCs to provide this range of services there is a requirement for an efficient and effective interprofessional team to work collaboratively to enable the local priorities to be met. The SSCCs interprofessional team may include:

- Social workers
- Health visitors
- Midwives
- Early years practitioners
- Nursery workers
- Administrative assistant
- Family nurse
- Job advisor
- Community outreach assistant

- Speech and language therapist
- Family support workers
- Play workers
- School nurse
- Centre manager
- Receptionist
- Children's workers
- Community liaison officer
- General practitioner

**NB** The list of professionals included in this list is by no means exhaustive as the professionals included in a SSCC vary from centre to centre. The members are not listed in any specific order.

The agencies involved in providing the services to SSCCs may include:

**Public Providers**

- Childcare
- Social care
- Health services
- Jobcentre Plus
- Adult education services
- Children's information services
- Housing support services

**Voluntary and Private Providers**

- Childcare
- Centre management service providers
- Community outreach organizations
- Ethnic support groups and refugee organizations
- Business and regeneration support agencies
- Housing support services

*Sure Start Children's Centres (National Audit Office, 2006)*

The large interprofessional team and the large number of agencies involved in the delivery of SSCCs show how complex this initiative is and to a greater or lesser extent the success of SSCCs depends on the success of how well these teams work interprofessionally and how fully the services are integrated.

## EVIDENCE BASE

Read the following articles to find out how successful the integration of services and interprofessional working has been in Sure Start Children's Centres:

- Edgley, A. and Avis, M. (2007) The perceptions of statutory service providers of a local Sure Start programme: a shared agenda? *Health and Social Care in the Community*, **15**(4): 379–386.

- Malin, N. and Morrow, G. (2007) Models of interprofessional working within a Sure Start 'Trailblazer' Programme. *Journal of Interprofessional Care,* **21**(4): 445–457.

- MacNeill, V. (2009) Forming partnerships with parents from a community development perspective: lessons learnt from Sure Start. *Health and Social Care in the Community,* **17**(6): 659–665.

## 2. Stroke

Stroke is one of the top three causes of death in the UK and around 300 000 people are living with moderate to severe disabilities as a result of stroke. Approximately 110 000 strokes and 20 000 transient ischaeamic attacks (TIA) occur in England each year. Without preventative action, there is likely to be an increase in strokes as the population ages (National Audit Office, 2010).

The *National Service Framework for Older People* (Department of Health, 2001a) sets out eight national standards and service models of care regarding health and social care services for older people. The NSFs were developed following the publication of the White Paper, *A First Class Service: Quality in the New NHS* (Department of Health, 1998b). The NSF for older people was developed in partnership with older people and their carers, health and social care professionals, NHS and social services managers and partner agencies. Standard five of the NSF for older people refers to stroke. The aim of this standard is to reduce the incidence of stroke in the population and to ensure that those who have a stroke have prompt access to integrated stroke-care services. The Standard is as follows:

- the NHS will take action to prevent strokes, working in partnership with other agencies where appropriate
- people who are thought to have had a stroke have access to diagnostic services, are treated appropriately by a specialist stroke service and subsequently their carers participate in a multidisciplinary programme of secondary prevention and rehabilitation.

Although Standard five of the NSF has on-going relevance and is still clinically valid, it is now the subject of a specific policy, the *National Stroke Strategy* (Department of Health, 2007b). The National Stroke Strategy is a ten-year vision, which defines markers for high quality stroke care, and sets out actions and progress measures. Collaboration between health and social care practitioners is key to the success of this strategy.

To encourage interprofessional working and the development of a seam-less care pathway for patients who have suffered a stroke, the support for stroke care has been divided into twenty-eight Stroke Care Networks across England. Each Stroke Care Network encompasses the whole stroke pathway by connecting different organizations and teams involved along the patient's journey, so individuals experience co-ordinated management from the first contact which extends to lifelong support as a stroke survivor. Networks involve stroke survivors and carers as active partners in coordinating and supporting service development (Department of Health, 2007b).

Also as part of the National Stroke Strategy, NHS Improvement – Stroke was set up to provide national support for improving stroke and TIA services. This was set up to provide support for, and work closely with, the stroke care networks. The following case study shows how the service for stroke patients can be improved by health and social care professionals working together.

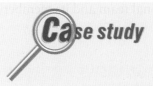

## Case study

### Lewisham integrated stroke project

In this project, colleagues across health and social care in South East London worked together to improve the service for stroke patients on transition from hospital to home and after they had left hospital. At the project outset, a typical Lewisham stroke patient would need to pass through up to seven different teams, with variations in the quality of service throughout. The average length of hospital stay was 22.5 days, which impacted on the number of acute stroke patients who could be admitted to the ward. Only 41 per cent of stroke patients spent more than 90 per cent of their stay on the stroke ward and the wait for generic community rehabilitation after hospital discharge was often greater than 12 weeks.

Through engagement with senior management and clinical staff and consultation with service users, bottlenecks in the transfer of care and rehabilitation process were identified and a collaborative approach across health, social care and voluntary organizations used to aspire to best practice. The pathway was re-designed, there was a focus on joint working and systems of communication and a reconfiguration of the workforce to include some new therapy posts and new ways of working and to integrate provision of stroke rehabilitation from several teams into a single integrated team.

A number of key improvements were made at ward level, including simplifying the discharge process, addressing inaccuracies of coding and implementing a key worker system. A pilot neuro-rehabilitation team was formed as part of the new integrated care team to address the lack of stroke specific community rehabilitation.

Service level agreements were re-negotiated with the third sector for family support at home and there was improved integration with social care staff and processes.

As a result, there is now a re-designed, more efficient, simplified stroke pathway in place and enhanced joint working with social care. Coordination of care has been improved with a more personalized holistic service. The length of stay has decreased to 19 days (March 2010) which has had an impact on the stroke Vital Sign with more than 80 per cent of stroke patients spending 90 per cent of their time on the stroke unit. The improvements made a significant impact on access to community waiting times for therapy falling by ten days or more for some therapies, even before the planned early supported discharge team was in place.

Referenced from *Improving Stroke Care, NHS Improvement – Stroke,* 2010 (Available in the public domain. Accessed June 2012)

There are three strands to an integrated stroke service:

- stroke prevention for those at risk of a first or further stroke
- specialist stroke services providing acute care and rehabilitation
- long-term support for stroke patients and their carers.

In this section, we will primarily focus on strands two and three of the integrated stroke service, discussing the interprofessional approach taken to stroke care. Strand two refers to the development of specialist stroke services. It is recognized that the outcomes for stroke patients are better when they are cared for by a specialist stroke team, within a dedicated acute and rehabilitation stroke unit. The key components of the specialist stroke service include:

- a specialist stroke team
- an acute stroke unit
- a stroke rehabilitation unit.

The specialist stroke team is a large interprofessional team and its membership typically includes:

- Stroke physician
- Stroke nurse consultant
- Occupational therapists
- Nursing staff
- Pharmacists
- Stroke-care coordinator
- Clinical psychologist
- Physiotherapist
- Social worker
- Speech and language therapist
- Community neuro-rehabilitation team.

The specialist stroke-care team working within a specialist acute and rehabilitation stroke unit will offer an integrated stroke service, as follows:

- The service will provide patient-focused care
- It will be ensured that the specialist stroke team will assess each patient as soon as they are admitted to hospital with a stroke
- The team will hold **Multidisciplinary Team (MDT)** meetings each week. At the MDT meeting, each patient will be discussed in detail, which gives all the members of the team an opportunity to understand the current progress in all aspects of their patients' care. The MDT meeting also enables the future care and treatment of patients to be discussed, planned and agreed (see Chapter 5 for further details on MDT meetings.)
- Carers and family members will be encouraged to participate in care right from the start. This enables more effective communication with the family and carers and facilitates the setting of realistic goals.

**Multidisciplinary Team (MDT)**
A group of people of different professions who meet on a regular basis to discuss individual patients. Each different professional contributes independently to the diagnostic treatment or care decisions regarding each patient case

As we can see, the specialist stroke team is an excellent example of an interprofessional team working and learning together to provide a quality service to stroke patients and their family and carers. The specialist stroke team does not, however, work in isolation and once the patient leaves the rehabilitation stroke unit, their care continues in the community. The rehabilitation services offered in the community are wide and varied and include:

- Day-care social services
- Dietetics
- Musculoskeletal physiotherapy
- Speech and language therapy

- District nursing service
- Wheelchair services
- Social-care occupational therapy services
- Leisure centre.

The voluntary sector is an important part of the interprofessional team caring for patients who have suffered a stroke and their family and carers. The Stroke Association, for example, is the major stroke charity in the UK that offers a wide range of services to those affected by stroke, including a Carer Support service, Communication Support service, Stroke Prevention Service, Getting Back to Life service and Information, Advice and Support service. The Stroke Association also works closely with statutory health and social services organizations to reduce the impact of stroke. For example, the Stroke Association produces information and resources for health and social care professionals working with those affected by stroke (The Stroke Association, 2012).

Other voluntary associations that work with those affected by stroke include:

- **Different Strokes.** This is run by and for younger people who have had strokes
- **Connect – the Communication Disability Network.** This organization works with people living with stroke and aphasia
- **Speakability.** This is a national charity that supports people living with aphasia and their carers.

> **aphasia**
> Is the loss of the ability to use and understand language; it can be speaking, writing or listening. It is usually caused by stroke, brain disease or injury

## EVIDENCE BASE

Go to the following websites and read about the services that these organizations provide for those affected by stroke:

- The Stroke Association **www.stroke.org.uk**
- Different Strokes **www.differentstrokes.co.uk**
- Connect – the Communication Disability Network **www.ukconnect.org**
- Speakability **www.speakability.org.uk**.

Education is a key factor in all aspects of stroke-care provision and interprofessional education is essential to ensure that high quality care and services is provided for people with stroke or at risk of stroke. A key principle of the *National Stroke Strategy* (Department of Health, 2007b) is to ensure that there is an appropriately stroke skilled workforce to meet the needs of patients. As we have discussed stroke services function in multidisciplinary teams and it is necessary to provide the stroke team staff with necessary skills and competencies, even if outside of traditional roles. For example, speech and language therapy staff training non-speech and language therapy colleagues in swallowing screening can provide much needed additional flexibility to the team. A Stroke Specific Educational Framework has been developed to help this process by providing a clear and structured description of patient need and associated clinical skills (Department of Health, 2009).

The interprofessional environment within which stroke care is offered provides an ideal interprofessional learning opportunity. In some specialist stroke units, monthly interprofessional education symposiums or journal clubs have been established. The specialist stroke teams are also responsible for developing and providing education programmes both within the hospital and in the community setting for members of the general public. Programmes include, for example, learning about stroke and stroke prevention. Often these programmes will be supplemented by written information.

This discussion has illustrated the impact that health and social care policies have had on the care provided to those people who have suffered a stroke and their family and carers. The development of an integrated stroke service has meant that a wide range of health and social care professionals are now committed to interprofessional working and learning and are collaborating effectively to provide a patient-focused service.

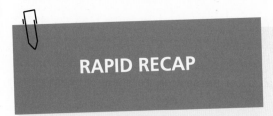

## RAPID RECAP

Check your progress so far by working through each of the following questions.

1 What are the five drivers for interprofessional working?

2 What three factors are still inhibiting successful interprofessional working?

3 What was the purpose of developing Sure Start?

4 What are the main Department of Health policies that have impacted on the delivery of stroke services in the UK?

If you have difficulty with more than one of the questions, read through the section again to refresh your understanding before moving on.

# REFERENCES

Asthana, A (2010) Sure Start children's centres told to charge for some services. *The Observer,* 14 December cited in Lloyd, N. and Harrington, L. (2012) The challenges to effective outcome evaluation of a national, multi-agency initiative: The experience of Sure Start. *Evaluation* **18** (1): 93–109.

The Beveridge Report (1942) *Social Insurance and Allied Services.* London: His Majesty's Stationery Office. Available from: http://www.nationalarchives.gov.uk. Accessed December 2012.

Crawford, K. (2012) *Interprofessional collaboration in social work practice.* London: Sage Publications.

Department for Education and Employment (1999) *Sure Start. Making a difference for children and families.* London: DfEE Publications.

Department for Education and Skills (2004) *Every child matters: change for children.* London: The Stationery Office.

Department of Health (1968) Report of the committee on local authority and allied personal social services (The 'Seebohm Report'), London: HMSO.

Department of Health (1989a) *Working for patients.* London: Department of Health.

Department of Health (1989b) *Caring for people: community care in the next decade and beyond.* London: Department of Health.

Department of Health (1997) *The new NHS, modern – dependable.* London: HMSO.

Department of Health (1998a) *Modernizing social services: promoting independence, improving protection, raising standards.* London: HMSO.

Department of Health (1998b) *A first class service: quality in the new NHS.* London: HMSO.

Department of Health (1998c) *National Service Frameworks.* London: Health Service Circular 1998/074.

Department of Health (1999a) *Health Act 1999 – modern partnerships for people.* London: HMSO.

Department of Health (1999b) *Agenda for change: modernizing the NHS pay system.* London: HMSO.

Department of Health (1999c) *Primary Care Trust (PCT's): establishing better services.* London: HMSO.

Department of Health (1999d) *Saving Lives: Our Healthier Nation:* London: Department of Health.

Department of Health (2000) *The NHS Plan: a plan for investment, a plan for reform.* London: HMSO.

Department of Health (2001a) *National service framework for older people.* London: HMSO.

Department of Health (2001b) *Health and social care Act 2001.* London: HMSO.

Department of Health (2004a) *National service framework for children, young people and maternity services.* London: HMSO.

Department of Health (2004b) *The NHS improvement plan: putting people at the heart of public services.* London: HMSO.

Department of Health (2004c) *Choosing health: making healthy choices easier.* London: HMSO.

Department of Health (2006) *Our health, our say, our care: a new direction for community services.* London: HMSO.

Department of Health (2007a) *Local involvement networks (LINks) explained.* London: HMSO.

Department of Health (2007b) *National stroke strategy.* London: HMSO.

Department of Health (2008a) *High quality care for all: NHS next stage review.* London: HMSO.

Department of Health (2008b) *High quality workforce: NHS next stage review.* London: HMSO.

Department of Health (2008c) *Health and social care Act, 2008.* London: HMSO.

Department of Health (2009) *Stroke-specific education framework.* London: Department of Health.

Department of Health (2010a) *Equity and excellence: liberating the NHS.* London: HMSO.

Department of Health (2010b) *A vision for adult social care: capable communities and active citizens.* London: HMSO.

Department of Health (2012) *The health and social care Act 2012.* London: HMSO.

Department of Health and Social Security (1974) *Report of the committee of enquiry into the care and supervision provided in relation to Maria Colwell.* London: HMSO.

Department of Health and Social Security (1990) *National Health Service & community care Act.* London: HMSO.

Edgley, A. and Avis, M. (2007) The perceptions of statutory service providers of a local Sure Start programme: a shared agenda. *Health and Social Care in the Community* 15(4): 379–386.

Healthcare Inspectorate Wales (2009) *Report of a review in respect of Mr D and the provision of mental health services, following the homicide of Father Paul committed in March 2007.* Available from www.hiw.org.uk.

HM Treasury (1998) *Cross-departmental review of provision for young children.* London: HMSO.

Hopkins, G (2007) What have we learnt? Child death scandals since 1994. Available at: http://www.communitycare.co.uk http://www.ccinform.co.uk/articles/2007/09/13/516/what+have+we+learned+child

+death+scandals+since+1944.html. Accessed June 2012.

Home Office (1945) Report by Sir William Monckton KCMG KCVO MC KC on the circumstances which led to the boarding out of Dennis and Terence O'Neill at Bank Farm, Minsterly and the steps taken to supervise their welfare, etc. Cmd 6636 London: Home Office.

Laming, Lord (2003) *The Victoria Climbié inquiry*. London: The Stationery Office.

Laming, Lord (2009) *The protection of children in England: a progress report*. London: The Stationery Office.

Malin, N. and Morrow, G. (2007) Models of interprofessional working within a Sure Start 'Trailblazer' programme. *Journal of Interprofessional Care*. **21** (4): 445–457.

National Audit Office (2006) *Sure Start Children's Centres*. London: The Stationery Office.

National Audit Office (2010) *Progress in improving stroke care*. London: The Stationery Office.

Secretary of State for Health (2001) *Learning from Bristol*. London: The Stationery Office.

Seebohm, F (1968) *Report of the Committee on Local Authority and Allied Personal Social Services*. London: HMSO.

Smith, J. (2002) The Shipman Inquiry: First Report. London: HMSO. Accessed June 2012.

Stroke Association available at: http://www.stroke.org.uk/ Accessed November 2012

Sure Start Unit (2001) *Sure Start: a guide to planning and delivering Sure Start*. London: Sure Start Unit.

Tope, R. and Thomas, E. (2007) *Health and social care policy and the interprofessional agenda*. Available from http://www.caipe.org.uk/silo/files/cipw-policy.pdf. Accessed June 2012.

Torbay Safeguarding Children Board (2010) *Serious Case Review*. Available from www.torbay.gov.uk/c18-execsumm.pdf.

World Health Organization (1978) *Alma Ata 1978 Primary Care*. Geneva: World Health Organization.

Younghusband, E. L. (1959) *Report of the working party on social workers in the local authority health and welfare services*. London: HMSO.

# CHAPTER 3

# TEAMS, TEAMWORK AND TEAM DYNAMICS

## LEARNING OBJECTIVES

*By the end of this chapter you should be able to:*

- Describe and define the different types of team

- Identify what helps and hinders effective teamwork

- Discuss the potential benefits of working in an interprofessional team

- Understand the key criteria for evaluating the effectiveness of teams.

## TEAMS AND TEAMWORK

The need for teams and effective teamwork within and between the health and social care sectors is crucial to improving the productivity of health and social care professionals and the quality of care that they provide.

The concept of teams and teamwork features prominently within the literature on interprofessional working. The definition of a team and teamwork are often taken for granted, but these terms mean different things to different people. It is therefore important when you are developing a team to find out what the other team members' views of what a team and teamwork are and how they value team working.

## What is a team?

Within the literature relating to teams and teamwork there are many differing definitions of a team. Two examples of attempts to define a team are given below:

> *A team is a small number of people with complementary skills who are committed to a common purpose, performance goals and approach for which they hold themselves mutually accountable.*
>
> *Katzenbach and Smith (1993, p. 45)*

> *A team is a group with a sense of common goal or task, the pursuit of which requires collaboration and the coordinations of the activities of its members, who have regular and frequent interactions with one another.*
>
> *Martin et al. (2010)*

If these two definitions along with the many others found within the literature are examined, the essential characteristics of a team emerge. Let us now consider what these 'essential' features of a team are. A team is a group of people who:

- share a common purpose and common goals
- have a clear understanding of each other's roles and abilities
- are task oriented and have different, but complementary skills
- have a shared knowledge, skills and resource base, and collective responsibility for the outcome of their decisions.

When considering an interprofessional team one further characteristic needs to be added to the above list of 'essential' characteristics:

- composed of persons from differing professions and/or organizations who work together to benefit the patient and their significant others.

## WHAT IS TEAMWORK?

The literature relating to teamwork reveals many definitions of teamwork. Two examples are given below:

> *Co-ordinated action carried out by two or more individuals jointly, concurrently or sequentially. It implies common agreed goals, clear awareness of, and respect for others' roles and functions. On the part of each member of the team, adequate human and material resources, supportive co-operative relationships and mutual trust, effective leadership, open, honest and sensitive communications, and provision for evaluations.*
>
> *Kekki (1990)*

> " *A dynamic process involving two or more health professionals with complementary backgrounds and skills, sharing common health goals and exercising concerted physical and mental effort in assessing, planning or evaluating patient care. This is accomplished through interdependent collaboration, open communication and shared decision-making. This in turn generates value-added patient, organizational and staff outcomes.*
>
> *Xyrichis and Ream (2008, p. 238)*

If we review the definitions of teamwork, recurrent themes can be identified. These can provide us with the essential characteristics of teamwork. Teamwork involves:

- having a common purpose and common objectives
- delegation and empowerment
- different professional contributions
- having systems in place to facilitate effective communication
- coordination, cooperation and joint thinking
- focusing on the patient to provide the best means of serving patient/client interests
- allowing team members to carry out the team's work and to manage itself as an independent group of people.

## EVIDENCE BASE

Read the following article to help you understand the concept of teamwork in the health and social care setting.

- Xyrichis, A. and Ream, E. (2008) Teamwork: a concept analysis. *Journal of Advanced Nursing* **61** (2): 232–241. Available from: **https://www.cihc.ca/library/bitstream/10296/407/1/XyrichisReam_Teamwork_Sep2007.pdf**
- After you have read the article, think about a team you are part of and consider how effective teamwork could be promoted to achieve a quality outcome for the patient.

## How does a team develop?

When a team is developing it will usually go through a series of stages before becoming really effective. It is useful to know the stages in team development, so that when your team appears to be going nowhere or members of the team are constantly arguing, you understand that this is normal! Understanding the stages will enable you to work towards moving the team on to the next stage.

Five stages of team development have been identified. They are forming, storming, norming, performing and adjourning (Tuckman and Jenson, 1977).

## Forming

When a team is forming, the team members spend time getting to know each other and individual team members avoid controversy, due to wanting to be accepted by the team. Team members may feel anxious because they do not know how the group will work or what exactly will be required of them.

During this stage the team members define the common objectives of the team and discussion centres on how the team are going to tackle achieving the agreed objective.

For the team to move from this stage to the next, team members must give up the comfort of safe, non-threatening topics and risk the possibility of conflict.

## Storming

As the name of this stage suggests, this is the time when things within the team may get stormy. Team members test each other, they question values and behaviours, the worth and feasibility of the common objectives may be challenged, as well as who is responsible for what. The guidance and direction of the leader may also be challenged. As a result of the discomfort generated by the conflict some members may withdraw and remain completely silent, while others may attempt to dominate.

If storming is not allowed to happen the team may never perform effectively. Storming is a healthy process in which the team evolves with a common set of values, believes and objectives.

In order to move from this stage to the next, team members must move from testing each other and conflict to 'listening to each other and problem solving'. Some teams never get beyond the storming stage in their development and may disintegrate because conflict between the team members cannot be resolved.

## Norming

During this stage the team starts to function harmoniously and individuals in the team value the differences that other members bring to the team. Team members are more willing to change their preconceived ideas or opinions on the basis of facts presented to them by other team members and members actively ask questions of one another.

Creativity is high during this stage with team members sharing feelings and ideas, asking and giving feedback to one another and exploring activities related to the common objectives of the team. Cooperation and collaboration replace the conflict and mistrust felt by the team members during the stormy stage of development.

Some teams do not go beyond the norming stage of development.

## Performing

When a team successfully reaches the performing stage, it will be working effectively and efficiently together to meet the team's common objectives. The team is now at its most productive, with the team and individual team members learning and developing together.

The performing stage can lead into a return to the forming stage if the team membership changes or to the final stage of development, adjourning.

## Adjourning

This stage marks the end of the working life of the team, with the team successfully reaching its common objectives and its work completed. The dismantling of a team can create a minor crisis for individual team members with team members feeling sad, nostalgic and 'mourning' the end of a team. The most effective interventions during the adjourning stage are those that help the team to tie up loose ends.

Although all teams pass through these five stages during their development, all teams develop at their own pace and in their own unique way. These stages may be longer or shorter for each team, or for individual members of the team. The formation of teams also differs; some teams can be represented as a spiral, while other teams form with sudden movements forward and then have periods of no change.

Health- and social-care teams are complex and dynamic and while the professional groups that make up the team normally remain fairly static, the individuals representing each profession may change on a more frequent basis. As a result, team development is not a straightforward linear process and the addition of new team members may cause the team to go back to the forming stage. Team development is likely to be 'stop-start' rather than a smooth development. It is important to recognize that new team members will not always result in the team going back to the forming stage; the team may stay at the same stage or may go back to the storming or norming stage of development dependent on the stage of team development reached before the new member joins the team. New team members will, however, always affect the dynamics of the team that they are joining. The impact of a new member on the team is not necessarily negative of course, and may be beneficial to the continuing development of the team.

## Reflective activity

Think of a team that you have recently been involved with and use the questions below to help you reflect on your team's development.

### 1  Forming

- What were the common objectives of the team?
- Did you all share the same expectations of the common objectives?
- Did you all have the same attitude to working in the team?
- Did you feel any anxiety on joining the team?

### 2  Storming

- Was there any conflict in the team?
- Did you all agree on how to tackle the common objectives?
- Was the authority of the team leader challenged?
- Did any team members withdraw from the team?

### 3  Norming

- Were the team members willing to change their preconceived ideas/opinions?
- Did you feel able to ask for and give constructive feedback to other team members?
- Did you cooperate with each other?
- Did you work out how to proceed?

### 4  Performing

- Did you work effectively and efficiently?
- Did the team focus on achieving the common objectives?
- Did you experience a sense of achievement?

### 5  Adjourning

- Did the team stop abruptly and you all go your own separate ways or did you successfully achieve the common objectives and go off together and socialize?
- Did you talk about the team and your experience of it?
- What sort of issues did you discuss or think about after the team dismantled?

# What types of people are in teams?

When considering interprofessional teams it is important to understand what an individual brings to a team. This will enable you to reflect on your preferred team role, the roles that other team members may take on and the impact that these roles have on both your behaviour towards others and the behaviour of others towards you.

Benne and Skeats (1948, cited in Payne, 2000) were some of the earliest writers to describe team roles. They divided team roles into three types:

- those roles involving task functions
- those roles involving maintenance functions
- those roles involving the individual.

## Roles involving task functions

These roles emphasize getting the job done and relate to the common objectives of the team (Table 3.1).

| Table 3.1   Roles involving task functions | |
|---|---|
| Initiator | Proposes new ideas, new tasks, new methods |
| Information-giver | Gives or volunteers to find out information |
| Clarifier | Takes individual contributions and clarifies; encourages people to be specific |
| Coordinator | Helps pull ideas and themes together |
| Evaluator | Critically evaluates ideas, proposals and plans |
| Summarizer | Summarizes what has been achieved |
| Questioner | Asks fundamental questions about the common objectives and challenges assumptions |

## Roles involving team maintenance

These roles emphasize keeping the team working together in harmony, dealing with conflict and issues of team maintenance (Table 3.2).

| Table 3.2   Roles involving team maintenance | |
|---|---|
| Encourager | Offers praise and agreement with other members; warm and understanding |
| Harmonizer | Mediates conflict and disagreements that occur |
| Compromiser | Seeks a compromise that all parties can accept |
| Standard setter | States or applies team standards |
| Gate keeper | Encourages others to participate; limits lengthy contributions |
| Team observer – commentator | Feeds back interpretations of team process |

## Roles involving the individual

These roles relate to the personality of the individual. Whilst these roles do not enhance teamwork, it is important for individual team members to recognize these personalities. If individual team members do not pay attention to these individual personalities it may result in the team working less efficiently and effectively (Table 3.3).

| Table 3.3   Roles involving the individual | |
| --- | --- |
| Aggressor | Attacks or criticizes; deflates others' status |
| Blocker | Negative; disagrees without reason |
| Dominator | Exerts authority; interrupts |
| Self confessor | Expresses irrelevant personal feelings to receive attention |
| Help seeker | Seeks sympathy through expressing insecurity or confusion |
| Playboy | Cynical; lack of involvement |
| Special-interest pleader | Masks own biases through pleading on behalf of others |
| Recognition seeker | Seeks attention; seeks important roles |

Since Benne and Skeats (1948, cited in Payne, 2000) identified the different types of roles found within a team, numerous teamwork writers have adapted their typology. However, the three roles related to task, team maintenance and the individual have remained.

Although Benne and Skeats' (1948, cited in Payne 2000) work has been significant, it is important when using these team roles to remember the following:

- the role descriptors describe patterns of behaviour within a team and not necessarily particular people or personality types
- an individual can adopt different roles at different times and in different situations, depending on the skills of the other team members
- team members may take on helpful and unhelpful roles at the same time.

It was not until the early 1980s that a completely new approach was taken to defining team roles. This work was undertaken by Dr Meredith Belbin, whose research examined the roles taken within the work tasks that a team undertake. Belbin's (1981) work originated from a management training exercise, in which over 200 simulated teams were set up to carry out tasks in groups. Following many years of research, nine roles were identified, which were considered necessary if a team was to be successful. These roles are set out in Table 3.4.

Belbin (1981) clustered these nine team-role types into three groups:

1 **Action-oriented roles** – Shaper, Implementer and Completer-finisher
2 **People-oriented roles** – Coordinator, Teamworker and Resource-investigator
3 **Cerebral roles** – Plant, Monitor Evaluator and Specialist.

| Table 3.4 | Belbin's team roles | | |
| --- | --- | --- | --- |
| **Role** | **Personality traits** | **Contributions** | **Possible weaknesses** |
| Implementer | Methodical<br>Practical<br>Conscientious<br>Reliable | Turns ideas into practical actions | Inflexible<br>Conservative<br>Lacks imagination<br>Does not inspire or motivate others |
| Shaper | Challenging<br>Dynamic<br>Thrives on pressure<br>Opportunistic | Driving force<br>Makes things happen<br>Galvanizes team | Impatient<br>Offends people's feelings<br>Argues or disagrees |
| Plant | Creative<br>Clever<br>Loner<br>Radical<br>Original<br>Unorthodox | Produces imaginative ideas<br>Solves difficult problems | Disregards practical details<br>Unrealistic<br>Can be isolated or become a scapegoat |
| Resource-investigator | Extrovert<br>Relaxed<br>Sociable<br>Communicative<br>Enthusiastic | Explores opportunities<br>Develops contacts<br>Good negotiator | Over-optimistic<br>Tendency to lose interest once initial enthusiasm has passed |
| Monitor evaluator | Judicious<br>Analytical<br>Prudent<br>Unemotional<br>Dispassionate | Judges accurately<br>Sees all options<br>Helps the team avoid mistakes | May appear dry, boring, over-critical<br>Lacks ability to inspire and motivate others |
| Teamworker | Cooperative<br>Diplomatic<br>Sympathetic<br>Sociable<br>Avoids conflict | Promotes harmony and team spirit<br>Averts disputes<br>Puts team before self | Indecisive in moments of crisis<br>Reluctant to do things that might hurt others |
| Completer-finisher | Painstaking<br>Anxious<br>Conscientious<br>Ordering | Dots the 'i's and crosses the 't's<br>Gives attention to detail<br>Delivers on time | Inclined to worry unduly<br>Has difficulty letting go or delegating work<br>Over-perfectionist |
| Coordinator | Mature<br>Confident<br>Good chairperson | Committed to team goals and objectives<br>Promotes decision-making<br>Delegates well | Can be seen as manipulative<br>Offloads personal work |
| Specialist | Single-minded<br>Self-starting<br>Dedicated<br>Committed | Provides knowledge and skills, which are in rare supply | Contributes only on a narrow front<br>Dwells on technicalities<br>Lacks interest in other people's subjects |

As with Benne and Skeat's work (1948, cited in Payne, 2000), Belbin's team role types should be used with caution. It is important to remember when a new team is developing that almost always people have a mix of roles and will have dominant and sub-dominant roles. Belbin's work provides a useful introduction to the idea of team roles, but its practical use in team building is limited.

More recent approaches to identifying team roles have focused on skills rather than personality types. For example, Margerison and McCann (1995) identified eight role preferences following discussions with successful teams. Table 3.5 identifies these role preferences.

| Table 3.5   Role preferences focusing on skills | |
|---|---|
| Creator–innovators | Independent people, who come up with ideas |
| Explorer–promoters | Sociable people, who bring ideas, contacts and resources |
| Assessor–developers | Practical people, who get ideas to work and test them against practical requirements |
| Thruster–organizers | Motivators, who organize people and systems |
| Concluder–producers | Consistent people, who maintain quality standards |
| Controller–inspectors | Careful people, who check and evaluate work |
| Upholder–maintainers | Stable people, who support others |
| Reporter–advisers | Patient people, who are good at collecting and presenting information |

Although recent analyses of team roles claim to focus on skills and not on personalities, it is apparent that many of the descriptors for team role types do have elements of personality styles within them. For example, in Table 3.5, explorer–promoters are described as 'sociable' people while upholder–maintainers are described as 'stable' people.

If we look back at the team role types described in this section, Benne and Skeats (1948, cited in Payne, 2000), Belbin (1981) and Margerison and McCann (1995), what is evident is that they bear remarkable similarities to each other. This would suggest that the research undertaken into team roles over the last 60 years has resulted in well-established categorizations of personalities from work and also that there is a consistent pattern of role division in the workplace.

Despite the criticisms levied at team role descriptors, this type of analysis can be useful to both the individual team member and the team. For the individual, being aware of their team role type provides an opportunity for professional development facilitating growth of the individual by learning new and additional roles to take up within the team. For the team, role analysis helps team members to see beyond defining other team members merely by their profession or job role.

It enables team members to identify and appreciate the wider contributions that they and other team members make to the team.

## Reflective activity

Think about two teams that you have been a member of in the last three months. One team should be an interprofessional work team and the other a team from your personal life. For each team consider the following points:

- List the dominant and sub-dominant team roles that you took up.
- Did you take up different dominant and sub-dominant team roles in each team?
- If so, why do you think that this happened?
- Using Belbin's model, identify the dominant team role that individual team members took up.
- Did each team have the nine team roles identified by Belbin? If so, was the team successful?

If your team had team roles missing, what impact did this have on the success of your teams?

## How are teams described?

Teams come in different shapes and sizes. There are small teams, large teams, temporary teams, permanent teams, real teams and virtual teams. There are multidisciplinary teams, cross-functional teams, problem solving teams and interprofessional teams. It is important that the distinctions between different types of team are understood, so that we know what type of team we are in and how we can develop the team to ensure that the team continues to meet the needs of specific patient groups and the requirements of the health and social care services.

The literature reveals that there are many different ways in which teams can be classified. Øvretveit's (1997) model for describing a team is particularly helpful because it relates specifically to interprofessional working in the health and social care sectors. This model puts forward four ways in which a team can be defined.

### Membership

It is important to agree who is in the team and who is not in the team and why. Øvretveit (1997) distinguishes between 'core' and 'associate' membership, the former usually referring to full-time membership and the latter referring to part-time membership.

The mix of different professions in a team and how many of each is in the team is another important consideration. If the mix of professions and the number of professionals is right then the skills of the team should match the individual needs of the patient.

The experience, status and seniority of the team membership must also be recognized to ensure that the experience that individuals bring to the team is valued. This is an important aspect of team membership, as this knowledge will help in matching team members with patients and will also help in determining individual team members' needs for professional development.

## Team process

A patient passes through a number of stages on their journey to and through a team. At each stage, decisions about the patient's care are made. The way in which the team makes these decisions reflects the type of team process that the team has adopted, and hence the patient pathway that the patient will follow. Øvretveit (1997) identifies six common types of team process: parallel pathway team; allocation team; reception-and-allocation team; reception-assessment-allocation-team; reception-assessment-allocation-review team; and hybrid-parallel-pathway team. Although the way in which a team makes decisions is different for each pathway, all the patients pass through the same stages in their care pathway:

Referral → Assessment → Care Plan → Review → Case closed

## Management structure

The management structure of a team that is, how the team is led and how the practitioners within that team are managed, is another way in which an interprofessional team can be described. Øvretveit (1997) identifies five team management structures.

**Profession-managed**  In this type of management structure, the members from each profession are separately managed by a manager from their own profession. In an interprofessional team, this may mean that members of the team are managed by separate agencies as well as separate departments. In a primary health care team, for example, team members may have managers from social services (if they are social workers), education (if they are special needs teachers) and from the health services (if they are nurses, physiotherapists or community midwives).

**Single manager**  In this case, team members from different professions are all managed by the same team manager (taken from one of the professions). In a single-manager structure, there may also be professional advisers to help the manager with professional issues.

**Joint management**  In this management structure, there is a team coordinator who organizes the work of the team, but each practitioner also relates to a manager from their own profession on professional issues.

**Team manager-contracted**  The team manager has a budget to buy services from professionally managed services.

**Hybrid management** As the name suggests this is a mixed management structure, with the team manager managing core staff, joint management responsibilities over other members of the team, and contracting in additional members to the team.

## Integration

Another way to describe a team is by considering the extent to which the team members are integrated into the team. The greater the degree of integration, then the closer the working relationship between the different professions within the team will be.

Katzenbach and Smith (1993) developed a model that differentiates between different types of team and different levels of performance according to a performance curve. This model is shown in Figure 3.1.

As Figure 3.1 illustrates, this model has five different types of team.

## Working group

This type of group shares information and best practices to make decisions to help each individual to function within their own area of responsibility. There are no common purpose or performance goals that require mutual accountability. There is little shared responsibility, with members usually only taking responsibility for their own results. Therefore, the focus is on individual performance. Working groups are found throughout health and social care organizations. The differences between work groups and teams are set out in Table 3.6.

| Table 3.6 Difference between work groups and teams | |
|---|---|
| **Work groups** | **Teams** |
| Individual accountability | Individual and mutual accountability |
| Efficient meetings with the main activity being to share information and perspectives | Open ended discussion and decision-making, problem solving, and planning |
| Focus on individual goals | Focus on team goals |
| Produce individual work products | Produce collective work products |
| Strong, clearly focused solo leader | Shared leadership roles |
| Skills are varied | Skills are complementary |
| Purpose, goals, approach to work shaped by manager | Purpose, goals, approach to work shaped by team leader with team members |

## Pseudo-team

A pseudo-team is one where the team members have no interest in agreeing a common goal for the team, but they still call themselves a team. In a pseudo-team, the sum of the whole is less than the potential of the individual parts. Pseudo-teams are often less effective than working groups because they have nothing concrete to do as a team that will contribute to the service/organization.

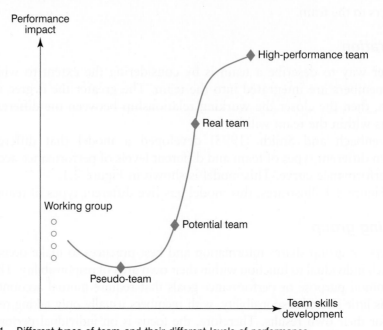

**Figure 3.1    Different types of team and their different levels of performance**
Adapted from *The Wisdom of Teams: Creating The High Performance Organization* by J. R. Katzenbach and D. K. Smith. Boston, MA. Copyright © 1993 by the Harvard Business School Publishing Corporation.

## Potential team

In a potential team the team members can see the need to improve performance. However, the team members require greater clarity about the purpose and goals of the team and need to work out a common approach. This form of teamwork is very common in organizations. The steepest performance gain comes between a potential and a real team.

## Real team

A real team is a small number of people with different but complementary skills, who are committed to a common purpose and common goals and who take collective responsibility for the outcome of their decisions. The performance impact of the real team is much greater than the potential team and working group.

## High-performance team

This type of team has all the characteristics of a real team but in addition it has team members who are committed to one another's personal growth, development and success. They far out-perform all other teams. Moving from a real team to a high performance team requires a very strong, personal commitment.

## *Reflective activity*

Think about an interprofessional team in which you are a member of the team. Using Øvretveit's (1997) model consider the following points:

● What type of interprofessional team are you in?

● Would the team be more effective if it operated as a different type of team? If so, what type of team?

● How do you think you could develop your team to enhance the services it provides to patients?

Using Katzenbach and Smith's (1993) model consider the following points:

● Where does your team sit on the curve?

● What does your team need to do to achieve its full potential?

## KEY POINTS

The advantages of interprofessional teams and teamworking are:

● A more responsive and patient-centred service

● Avoids duplication of work and fragmentation of the service

● More effective and efficient use of staff, which leads to more satisfying roles and career pathways for health and social care professionals

● A more effective service provision through improved organization and planning.

## What does an interprofessional team look like?

There are many examples of interprofessional teams working within the health and social care sector. Two examples of interprofessional teams that have developed significantly in recent years are primary health care teams and palliative-care teams.

### *Primary health care teams*

Primary health care has been defined by the World Health Organization declaration of Alma Ata as:

❝ *The first level contact of individuals, the family and the community with the national health system which brings health care as close as possible to where people live and work, and constitutes the first element of a continuing health process.*

*WHO (1978)*

| Table 3.7   Members of a primary health care team | |
|---|---|
| • General practitioners | • Diabetic specialist nurse |
| • Practice managers | • Occupational health nurses |
| • Practice nurses | • Audiologists |
| • Nurse practitioners | • Paramedics |
| • Community nurses | • Macmillan nurses |
| • Community midwives | • Community matrons |
| • Health visitors | • Health care assistants |
| • Occupational therapists | • Podiatry |
| • Social workers | • Community pharmacist |
| • Physiotherapists | • Stoma nurses |
| • Health trainers | • Art therapists |
| • Receptionists | • Falls prevention coordinator |
| • Administrative and clerical staff | • Dentists |
| • Private sector e.g. BUPA | • Residential and nursing homes |
| • Counsellors | • Opticians |
| • Voluntary agencies e.g. Age UK, Marie Curie Cancer Care, Carers Trust, Stroke Association | • School nurses |

**NB** The list of professionals included in this table is by no means exhaustive as the professionals included in a primary health care team vary from region to region. The members are not listed in any specific order.

A primary health care team can, therefore, be described as a group of professionals delivering health services in the community at the first point of contact with the health service. Table 3.7 indicates those health and social care professionals typically considered to form part of a primary health care team.

As Table 3.7 illustrates, a primary health care team is larger than the optimum team size of eight to ten members. If, however, the structure of the primary health care team is examined, it can be seen that different types of team are operating. There are large network structures, which include both health and social care professionals. Within these networks, communication tends to be intermittent and team members will network with each other as and when the need arises. More formally structured teams exist, which are based around general medical practices. These teams will be smaller with 10 to 15 members and communication will be tighter than that which occurs within the networks, although as with networks, communication will be broad. Finally, small individual **patient-centred** teams exist, which tend to be task based and time limited. Communication within these teams is frequent, full, but narrower, as it is focused on specific patient issues (Royal Pharmaceutical Society of Great Britain and the British Medical Association, 2000).

This range of different team types means that individuals could be contributing as members of different teams at different times, or even at the same time (see Figure 3.2).

**Patient-centred**
Making the patient the centre of the team's purpose

## Reflective activity

Think about your local primary health care team and consider the following points from both a professional and patient viewpoint:

● Which members of your primary health care team have you come into contact with?

● What types of primary health care teams did/do you come into contact with?

● Draw a diagram(s) to illustrate the different types of team and the team members that you have come into contact with.

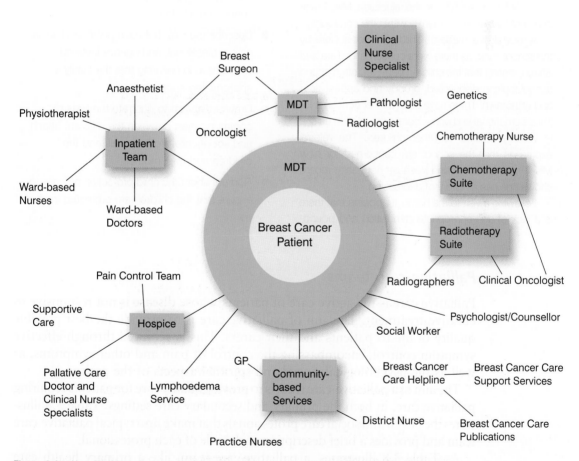

Figure 3.2   How health and social care teams might form around a patient with breast cancer
National Voices (Available in the public domain from: http://www.nationalvoices.org.uk/webs-care)

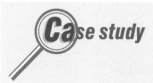

## A family in crisis

Miss Frank is 25 years old; she is a single mother to three children Tara (nine years old), Shaun (six years old) and Peter (three years old). She is currently eight months pregnant with her fourth child. Miss Frank has recently relocated following the breakdown of her abusive relationship with Peter's father, which led her to flee the relationship with her children. The family now live in a refuge. The children do not have any contact with their fathers and due to the relocation, Miss Frank does not have friends or family within the community.

A referral was made to Children's Social Care by the school nurse as there were concerns for Tara and Shaun, stating that the children bed-wet, often attend school looking dishevelled, grubby and appear tired and withdrawn. There have been further concerns for Tara's emotional and behavioural presentation as she is verbally abusive to other children. The referral expresses that the school are concerned for how Miss Frank is coping and because her health record shows she has a history of depression.

Following a visit to the home, it appears that there is a lack of age-appropriate stimulation and bound-aries set for the children. Tara appears to be the primary support for her mother, assisting in a variety of household tasks including assisting with childcare tasks. The children's bedrooms are bare and Shaun is sleeping on a mattress on the floor. Through the initial stages of the assessment it was also apparent that Peter is not toilet trained and his speech is delayed.

A large number of professionals, involved with the family include: a children's social worker, school nurse, teachers, health visitor, midwife, doctor's, mental health workers, Home-Start, Benefits agency, speech therapist and Children's Centre.

With reference to the case study:

- Discuss the type of team that is involved in supporting this family.

- Describe the role that each health and social care professional, and agency involved, would have in ensuring that the family is appropriately supported.

- Draw a diagram to illustrate the lines of communication between the different health and social care professionals and the children and their mother.

- Find out about the child protection process to ensure that the children are protected from harm.

## Palliative-care teams

Palliative care is the active care of patients whose disease is not responsive to curative treatment. The aim of palliative care is to provide the best possible quality of life to patients and their carers. This is achieved through effective symptom control, encompassing the control of pain and other symptoms, as well as the psychological, social and spiritual aspects of the patient.

The aim of a palliative-care team is to provide quality care for patients requiring palliative care, in both the primary and secondary care settings. Table 3.8 illustrates the health and social care professionals that make up a typical palliative-care team and provides a brief description of the role of each professional.

As Table 3.8 illustrates, a palliative-care team, like a primary health care team, is larger than the widely believed optimum size for a team to function effectively (eight to ten people). It may be more appropriate to call both these teams an enterprise, that is, a palliative-care enterprise and a primary health care enterprise.

**Enterprise**
A team with more than 40 members

If the structure of the palliative-care team is considered, it can be seen that, as with the primary health care team, different types of team are operating. The focus of these different types of team, as with any health- or social-care team, is the patient and their significant others. Thus, the health and social care professionals that make up the palliative-care team caring for a patient will depend on the type and progress of the disease, as well as the social and psychological care that the patient requires at any one point of time. This means that while there will be a 'core' team caring for a patient's palliative-care needs, the team will expand as and when appropriate. For example, if a patient with terminal breast cancer develops painful bony metastases in their thoracic vertebrae, they may be offered radiotherapy to control the pain. At this point, the palliative-care team caring for this patient would expand to include, for example, an oncologist, therapeutic radiographers and a Macmillan nurse. As this example illustrates, individual health- or social-care professionals will be members of different patient-centred care teams at the same time.

The primary health care team and palliative-care team are just two examples of interprofessional teams found in the health and social care sector. Both these examples demonstrate the complexity of interprofessional health and social care teams, providing some insight into the challenges that face professionals in working effectively as part of such a large, complex and changing team.

| Table 3.8 Members of a typical palliative-care team | | |
|---|---|---|
| **Place of care** | **Team** | **Role** |
| Community | Primary health care team with the addition of specialist palliative-care involvement as below <br> • Specialist palliative-care nurse | • Advises and provides support to the patient and their family and other professionals |
| | • Hospice-at-home | • This may be a stand-alone team or attached to a hospice or palliative-care team <br> • Provides clinical care and support, often in symptom management of end-of-life issues |
| | • Specialist palliative-care physician | • Provides advice and assessment in complex symptom management <br> • May visit the patient at home or may see the patient as an outpatient |
| | • Marie Curie nurses (Charitable Fund) | • Provide sitting and hands-on care for patients, as respite for main carer at end of life |

*(Continued)*

| Table 3.8   Members of a typical palliative-care team   (Continued) | | |
|---|---|---|
| **Place of care** | **Team** | **Role** |
| Hospital | Secondary health care team with the addition of:<br>● Specialist palliative-care physician and an attached team | ● Assesses and treats patients referred by other clinicians |
| | ● Specialist palliative-care nurse (often referred to as a Macmillan nurse) | ● Advise and provide support for the patient and their family and other professionals |
| | ● Oncology nurses | ● Provide advice and support to the patient and their family and other professionals on site-specific issues, for example breast, prostate or haematology problems |
| | ● Complementary therapists | ● Provide a range of therapies, massage, counselling |
| | ● Lymphoedema specialist nurse | ● Provides care and treatment for patients with lymphoedema |
| Hospice or hospice-at-home team | This is usually a charitable institution with varying amounts of money given by the local NHS Trusts.<br>The hospice team will include:<br>● Registered nurses<br>● Doctors<br>● Pharmacist<br>● Counsellor<br>● Occupational therapist<br>● Physiotherapist<br>● Social worker<br>● Chaplain<br>● Complementary therapist<br>● Art therapist<br>● Music therapist<br>● Lymphoedema specialist<br>● Dietician | The hospice or hospice-at-home team provide specialist support in the following:<br>● Physical care<br>● Social care<br>● Psychological care<br>● Spiritual care<br>● Domains of assessed care<br>● Symptom management of complex problems<br>● Specialist access to services due to end-of-life issues<br>● Family-support teams (specialist social workers) often deal with social/psychological issues, preparation for bereavement, loss and counselling<br>● Specialist complementay therapy, art, music, massage, aromatherapy |

*Health care professional*

Sam, an experienced adult nurse, talks of her experiences of attending ward rounds in a palliative care setting. Such rounds involve many members of the multidisciplinary team; namely the medical consultant, the nurse caring for the patient, physiotherapist, occupational therapist and a nurse from the homecare team. The patient is always the centre of care and relatives are invited to join the patient if this is their wish. This ensures good communication is achieved and everybody works collaboratively in the patient's best interests. Information is shared between the patient and all the disciplines and a holistic approach to care is taken. The nurse caring for the patient may act as the patient's advocate and ensures any questions the patient may have are answered.

It is really important that the patient does not feel overwhelmed by a ward round and this is generally achieved well in this setting by good non-verbal communication. The problems that may be encountered even when a round is performed well is that of a lack of privacy when patients are being cared for in a bay, conversations are audible by others through curtains. This can be overcome by moving to a quiet area, although this is not always achievable. Taking part in a well-performed ward round as a nurse who knows her patients well gives true job satisfaction.

## What makes an interprofessional team an effective team?

As we have already discussed, interprofessional teams come in many shapes and sizes within the health and social care sectors, from larger network teams through to smaller individual patient-centred teams. It is important that, whatever the shape and size of the team, the team is effective. The following factors contribute towards effective teamwork.

### Clear team goal

It is very difficult to get there if you do not know where you are going!

An effective team will have a shared common goal, which is clear and achievable, providing team members with a focus and direction for their efforts. The goal will have defined outcomes that are measurable, enabling team members to monitor their progress towards successful achievement of their overall goal.

### Open communication

Members of effective teams inform each other of who is doing what, when, where and how. Ensuring that relevant information is shared with each team member will enable the team to make the best decisions, thus enhancing the service that the team provide to their patients. Effective teams do not guard information; they share it freely.

## Support for innovation

Effective teams work in a climate in which innovation is encouraged and supported by their organization, with adequate time and resources factored in. Management support for innovation encourages teams to develop new ideas and ways in which to work that will ultimately enhance the morale and thus the output of the team. Research into the effectiveness of health care teams in the NHS (Borrill *et al.*, 2000) has found that teams comprising a mix of professional groups are linked to higher innovation than teams of one group.

## High levels of participation

All team members must participate fully in the team's activities if the team is to function well. For this to occur there must be a general climate of trust within the team. Team members should feel 'safe' to contribute ideas, and challenge current practices without fear of recrimination from other team members.

## Clear roles and responsibilities

Teams will work more effectively if the roles and responsibilities of team members are clearly articulated and understood by those team members. Misunderstandings and conflicts often occur when roles and expectations are not clearly defined. Awareness among the team of each other's roles and responsibilities will help teams to cope constructively with professional conflicts.

## Competent team members

Competent team members are crucial if a team is to work effectively. Equally important is that the team members are placed in the right position. Sometimes, a highly competent professional can be ill-placed, which can upset the team functioning. It is important that problems are dealt with and that if a team member is persistently failing to work with others and targets are not being met, that they are dealt with through the appropriate management and disciplinary procedures.

## Effective time management

How a team structures its meetings and meets its deadlines reflects its effectiveness. Teams that manage their meetings well encourage high performance and therefore they have an increased chance of meeting their goals.

## Values diversity

The members of an interprofessional health- or social-care team have diverse value systems which can be a key source of interpersonal conflict within a team. However, if a team learns to value each other's differences, they can build on each other's strengths. The overall impact is that individuals appreciate diversity and work together more effectively.

## High level of commitment

The effectiveness of a team is associated with a high level of commitment to quality in the team. Commitment to a team is only achieved through all members of the team sharing the same values. This will mean that team members will be motivated to achieve their goals through the provision of a high-quality, innovative service. Team members will enjoy their work, giving them job satisfaction, leading to organizational commitment.

## Joint education and training

Work-based learning enables practitioners to learn more effectively together (Manley *et al.*, 2009). If professionals are learning together, this will encourage and enhance effective interprofessional teamwork. Opportunities for interprofessional education occur at both pre- and post-registration level. The education and learning which may take place is varied: qualificatory courses offered by a university; local/national/ international joint conferences/study days; interprofessional training days offered by local service providers; continuing professional development in the practice environment linked to current health- or social-care initiatives.

## Effective conflict resolution

Effective teams expect conflicts and differences of opinion, but how the team resolve their conflicts can make or break them. An effective team will focus on the task at hand, not on the individuals in the team, which helps the team move forward and redirect their focus toward positive outcomes.

## Moral support and team spirit

Members of effective teams support each other, take pride in and feel loyalty for their teams. The team members will let each other know how they appreciate each other's efforts and ideas and will help each other as and when needed.

## *Reflective activity*

Working in teams can be rewarding, but at times it is difficult and frustrating. It is just as important to be aware of those factors that can result in a team under-performing as well as those factors that enhance teamwork. Table 3.9 below identifies some of the things that can go wrong in teams. Think about a team in which you are an active member. This could be a work-related team or a team you are involved with in your leisure time, for example a sports team or a musical band. Complete the table below by considering the following:

- Identify those problems which are present in your team and which you feel need most attention.
- For each problem identified, what action could you take to make your team a more effective team?

| Table 3.9    What might be going wrong? | | |
| --- | --- | --- |
| **Tick** | **What might be going wrong?** | **Action to be taken** |
| | Not listening to each other | |
| | Not clarifying what your objective is | |
| | Allowing individuals to dominate | |
| | Allowing individuals to withdraw | |
| | Not recording what has been decided | |
| | Not recognizing the feelings of members of the team | |
| | Blaming each other for not meeting deadlines | |
| | Not clarifying who is going to do what | |
| | Not clarifying what has to be done by when | |
| | Not contributing equally to the progress of the team | |
| | Not being committed to the team | |
| | Not managing team meetings well | |
| | Not keeping to agreed practices | |
| | Not generating new ideas | |

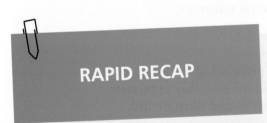

## RAPID RECAP

Check your progress so far by working through each of the following questions.

1  What are the essential features of a team?

2  What are the essential characteristics of teamwork?

3  What are the five stages of team development?

4  List Belbin's nine team roles, which he considered were necessary if a team was to be successful.

5  What factors contribute towards effective interprofessional teamwork?

If you have difficulty with more than one of the questions, read through the section again to refresh your understanding before moving on.

# REFERENCES

Belbin, R.M. (1981) *Management teams: why they succeed or fail*. London: Heinemann.

Borrill, C.S., Carletta, J., Carter, A.J., Dawson, J.F., Garrod, S., Rees, R., Richards, A., Shapiro, D. and West, M.A. (2000) *The effectiveness of health care teams in the National Health Service. Final report*. Available from: www.homepages.inf.ed.ac.uk/jeanc/DOH-final-report.pdf.

Katzenbach, J.R. and Smith, D.K. (1993) *The wisdom of teams: creating the high performance organization*. Boston, MA: Harvard Business School Press.

Kekki, P. (1990) *Teamwork in primary care*. Geneva: World Health Organization.

Manley, K., Titchen, A. and Hardy, S. (2009) Work based learning in the context of contemporary health care education and practice: a concept analysis. *Practice Development in Health Care* 8 (2): 87–127.

Margerison, C.J. and McCann, D. (1995) *Team management: practical new approaches* (2nd ed.). Oxford: Management Books.

Martin, V., Charlesworth, J. and Henderson, E. (2010) *Managing health and social care*, 2nd edition. Oxford: Routledge.

Øvretveit, J. (1997) How to describe interprofessional working. In *Interprofessional working for health and social care* (eds. Øvretveit,J., Mathias, P. and Thomson, T.). Macmillan: London, pp. 9–33.

Payne, M. (2000) *Teamwork in multiprofessional care*. Basingstoke: Palgrave.

Pritchard, P. and Pritchard, J. (1994) *Teamwork for primary and shared care: a practical workbook* (2nd edn). Oxford University Press: Oxford.

Royal Pharmaceutical Society of Great Britain and the British Medical Association (2000) *Teamworking in primary health care: realising shared aims in patient care. Final report*. Royal Pharmaceutical Society of Great Britain and BMA: London. Available from: www.rpsgb.org.uk/pdfs/teamworking.pdf.

Tuckman, B.W. and Jenson, M.A.C. (1977) Stages of small group development revisited. *Group and Organizational Studies*, 2: 419–427.

World Health Organization (1978) *Alma Ata 1978 Primary Care*. Geneva: World Health Organization.

Xyrichis, A. and Ream, E. (2008) Teamwork: a concept analysis. *Journal of Advanced Nursing* 61 (2): 232–241.

# CHAPTER 4

# LEADERSHIP AND EXPERTISE

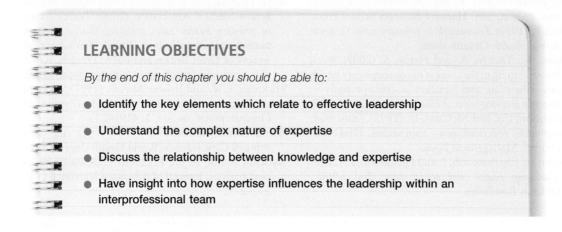

**LEARNING OBJECTIVES**

*By the end of this chapter you should be able to:*

● Identify the key elements which relate to effective leadership

● Understand the complex nature of expertise

● Discuss the relationship between knowledge and expertise

● Have insight into how expertise influences the leadership within an interprofessional team

## WHAT IS LEADERSHIP?

Leadership ...

" *Go to the people*
*Live among them*
*Start with what they have*
*Build with them*
*And, when the deed is done*
*The mission accomplished*
*The people will say*
*'We have done it ourselves'*

*Lao Tzu (6th century BC)*

Although leadership has been of interest to society for many years, there still appears to be no ultimately authoritative definition of leadership within the literature. Examples of definitions of leadership are given below:

" *Leadership is a process whereby an individual influences a group of individuals to achieve a common goal.*

*Northouse (2010, p. 3)*

> ❝ *Leaders ask questions to set direction, put the right people in the right positions, seek insight from all levels and ensure resources are allocated to the highest priority, while acting ethically at all times and engaging people to stretch beyond what is comfortable to maximize results.*
>
> *Cohen (2009, p. 16)*

> ❝ *Leadership is a process of motivating people to work together collaboratively to accomplish great things.*
>
> *Vroom and Jago (2007, p. 18)*

As well as the differing definitions of leadership, the literature reveals that leadership is a complex topic, with the existence of many theories and typologies. Trying to navigate your way through the wealth of literature on leadership could be likened to trying to find your way out of a maze!

The approach taken to leadership in this chapter will be to trace the developments in ideas of leadership and to discuss the significance of those developments to interprofessional leadership and interprofessional working.

Early research into leadership was concerned with identifying traits of leadership, so that the people with the right traits could be selected for leadership roles. The so-called 'trait theory' was based on the premise that leaders are born rather than created. Studies over the last sixty years (Stogdhill, 1974; Mann, 1959; Kirkpatrick and Locke, 1991; Zaccaro, Kemp and Bader, 2004) have identified a long list of traits and characteristics considered to be essential to a successful leader. From these studies five major traits emerge:

1 Intelligence
2 Self confidence
3 Determination
4 Integrity
5 Sociability

However, early researchers began to identify problems with the trait theory. For example, this approach did not look at whether the leaders were effective or not and it is also difficult to identify whether individuals have the required traits or not. As a result, researchers turned their attention to what leaders did, that is, how they behaved, especially towards their followers (team members). Researchers, therefore, moved from studying the leaders to studying leadership. There was recognition that leadership was a behavioural pattern that could be learned. Different patterns of behaviour were grouped together and labelled as leadership styles. The following section discusses these leadership styles.

## LEADERSHIP STYLES

A number of different leadership styles emerged from these studies, which were based on different assumptions and theories. The style that a leader adopts is based on their beliefs, values and preferences as well as the organizational cultures and norms around them. Different organizations will encourage some styles while discouraging others. The following leadership styles will be considered:

1 Participative leadership
2 Situational leadership
3 Transactional leadership
4 Transformational leadership
5 Charismatic leadership
6 Authentic leadership

## Participative leadership

A participative leader, as the name suggests, is a leader who actively involves other people in the decision-making process, for example, team members, peers, managers and appropriate stakeholders. The level of involvement that others have in the decision-making process will vary depending on the preferences and beliefs of the leader and the type of decision being made. (Table 4.1).

| Table 4.1   Spectrum of participation | | | | |
|---|---|---|---|---|
| **Not participative** | | | | **Highly participative** |
| Autocratic decision by leader | Leader proposes decision, listens to feedback and then decides | Team proposes decision, leader has final decision | Joint decision with team as equals | Full delegation of decision to team |

Advantages of this style of leadership include:

- team members are more committed to decisions if they have been involved in the decision-making process
- involvement in decision-making improves the team members' understanding of the issues involved
- team members deciding together make better decisions than one person alone.

Participative leadership is not without its critics and its main problem is one shared with the trait theory. Researchers often did not consider the context or setting in which the leadership style was being used. For example, advocates of participative leadership assumed that the same style of leadership would work as well in a team of footballers as in an accident and emergency department.

## Situational leadership

As researchers realized that both the environment and the abilities of the team members significantly influenced the style that the leader adopted, researchers began to turn their attention to these two factors. A number of models emerged which were based on the interaction of the characteristics of the leader, the characteristics of the followers and the situation. One of the more influential models that emerged is the one developed by Hersey and Blanchard (1977). See Figure 4.1.

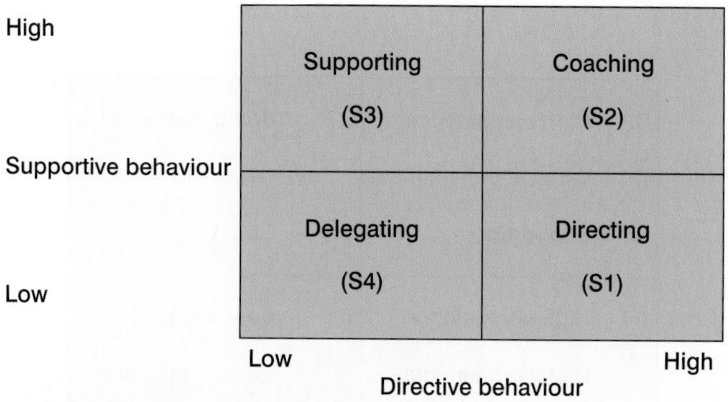

Figure 4.1   Hersey and Blanchard's four leadership styles

This model identified four leadership styles that could be selected to deal with contrasting situations. The style that the leader chose depended upon the amount and support that the leader needed to give to an individual team leader.

### Directing (S1)

The leader defines the roles and tasks of the team members and supervises closely. The leader makes the decisions and tells the team members, so communication is largely one way. This style of leadership might be used when a new member joins the team, or where a task has to be completed within a very short time span.

### Coaching (S2)

The leader still defines the roles and tasks, but seeks ideas and suggestions from the team member. The leader still makes the decision but communication is much more two way.

## Supporting (S3)

The leader gives day-to-day decisions to the team member. The leader facilitates and takes part in the decisions, but control is with the team member.

## Delegating (S4)

The leader is still involved in decisions and problem solving but the control is with the team member.

An effective leader will be versatile and will be able to move around the four leadership styles depending on the situation. There is no one right style but a leader will have a preferred style. As previously stated, the style adopted by the leader will not only depend on the situation but also on the characteristics of the individual team member. To take this into account, Hersey and Blanchard (1977) identified four development levels for individual team members, which, like the leadership styles, varied depending on the situation (see Figure 4.2). The four development levels are as follows:

| D3 | High competence | D2 | Some competence |
|----|-----------------|----|-----------------|
|    | Variable commitment | | Low commitment |
| S3 | Supporting | S2 | Coaching |
| D4 | High competence | D1 | Low competence |
|    | High commitment | | Low commitment |
| S4 | Delegating | S1 | Directing |

Figure 4.2   The relationship between the four leadership styles and the four development levels of the team member

- **D1** – Generally lacking the specific skills required for the task and lacks confidence and/or motivation.
- **D2** – May have some of the relevant skills, but will be unable to do the task without some support. The task or situation may be new to them.
- **D3** – Experienced and capable, but may lack confidence to do it without support or the motivation to do it well.
- **D4** – Experienced at the job/task and comfortable with their ability to do it well.

The key feature of a situational leadership model, like the Hersey and Blanchard (1977) model, is that if a leader selects a style that is suited to the context and to the ability of the team member, the leader and consequently the team will be more successful. There are, however, limitations with such a model which include:

- The model mainly focuses on the relationship between leaders and their team members and does not consider issues of organizational structure, politics, economics and professional socialization.

- The model does not take into account cultural factors. Cultural factors influence the way people carry out, and respond to, different leadership styles.

## Reflective activity

A senior practitioner joins your team and you are asked to look after him during his first few days.

With reference to this scenario, consider the following:

- think about what the senior practitioner needs to know/find out in the first few days in your team

- for each task identified, use Hersey and Blanchard's (1977) model to select the appropriate style of leadership

- think about the benefits and drawbacks for both you and your colleague of adopting the style of leadership that you have selected for each task.

## Transactional leadership

Transactional leadership is built on a system of give and take, with the relationship between the leader and the follower being developed from the exchange of rewards and promises for the effort put in by the follower, for example, salary increase, attendance at study days/conferences, recognition, praise. The leader clarifies goals and objectives, communicates and organizes tasks and activities for their team members to ensure that the specified goals of the team are met (Burns, 1978). This style of leadership is hierarchical and is a reactive, as opposed to proactive, style of leadership, in that it deals with day-to-day activities and issues. It has been found that this style of leadership is more evident in first-level managers, than in high-level managers (Avolio and Bass, 1988). A first-level manager would be a practitioner who is leading other practitioners in the day-to-day delivery of care to patients/clients. An example of a first-level manager would be a senior therapeutic radiographer, responsible for the day-to-day running of a treatment unit in an oncology department. The senior radiographer would have responsibilities including scheduling of patients, treatment delivery, ensuring that the team all have coffee and lunch breaks, and problem solving. As a first-level manager's primary role is operational rather than strategic, it is not surprising that first-level managers have a tendency to adopt a transactional style of leadership. First-level managers also usually work in an environment that is conducive to a transactional leadership style. Transactional leadership is often found in stable environments where there is no acute sense of impending crisis or major change. Until the late 1980s, when changes to the traditional ways of working started to happen within the UK, transactional leadership was common within the NHS with leaders and teams feeling that they 'knew where they stood'. Even in today's constantly changing NHS, transactional leadership still has its place, for example, a culture of 'following the rules' is known to be effective in areas such as planning, budgetary control and organizing (Barr and Dowding, 2012).

Despite much research that highlights the limitations of transactional leadership, this is a popular approach that is still used today.

Transformational and charismatic leadership styles are also currently popular. It is these leadership styles that are used in the leadership development programmes that are aimed at leaders working in the health sector. These two styles of leadership are discussed in the following two sections.

## Transformational leadership

Transformational leadership is concerned with improving the performance of followers and developing followers to their fullest potential. The foundation of transformational leadership rests on the four behaviours that were identified by Bass (1985). These four behaviours are also referred to as the four I's of transformational leadership:

1 idealized influence
2 inspirational motivation
3 intellectual stimulation
4 individual consideration

### Idealized influence (Northouse, 2010)

This describes leaders who act as strong role models for the team and team members wish to emulate them. The behaviours associated with idealized influence include:

- very high standards of moral and ethical conduct
- being counted on to do the right thing
- articulating a vision for the future which is exciting.

### Inspirational motivation (Northouse, 2010)

Behaviours associated with inspirational motivation include:

- inspiring the team members to become committed to and part of the shared vision in the organization
- communicating optimism about future goals

- encouraging followers to go beyond self-interest for the good of the group
- providing reassurance that obstacles can be overcome
- encouraging confidence in achieving and carrying out goals and tasks.

## Intellectual stimulation (Northouse, 2010)

This is characterized by encouraging intelligence, consistency, logical thinking and careful problem solving. The behaviours associated with intellectual stimulation include:

- actively seeking different perspectives when solving problems
- suggesting new ways of looking at completing tasks
- encouraging creativity and innovation
- encouraging rethinking of ideas that have not been questioned in the past.

## Individual consideration (Northouse, 2010)

Individual consideration is concerned with the leader treating the followers as individuals and not just as members of the group. Behaviours related to individual consideration include:

- spending time teaching and coaching
- using delegation to help individuals to grow through personal challenges
- actively listening to others' concerns.

If we put these four behaviour types together then we start to build a picture of what a transformational leader 'looks like'. Below is an account of what a transformational leader might look like and feel like for their followers.

A transformational leader is concerned with change and action, in other words they are visionary. They put passion and energy into everything they do and in doing so they engage the hearts and minds of others. This style of leadership requires facilitation and concern for the individual team members.

Transformational leaders develop a clear collective vision that will excite and enthuse their team members and they communicate it effectively to their team members. The leader takes every opportunity to 'sell' the vision to their team, encouraging team members to commit to the vision. Trust and personal integrity are central features of the relationship that the leader has with the followers. It is through the followers' trust and respect in their leader that the followers are motivated to perform beyond expectation (Bass and Avolio, 1994).

A transformational leader is always visible and by acting as role models, they inspire team members to put the good of the whole team above self-interest. The leader encourages team members to be more innovative and is prepared to take personal risk. It is the leader's unwavering commitment that keeps the team members going, particularly when the team begins to believe that the vision can never be achieved.

Transformational leaders coach and mentor team members, encouraging them to develop both personally and professionally. They care about individual team members and want them to succeed.

When the benefits of transformational leadership for the team are considered, it is perhaps not surprising that this style of leadership is frequently used in leadership development programmes within health and social care settings. The benefits of transformational leadership include:

- significant increases in team performance
- higher commitment to the team from individual team members
- increased trust in the leader from team members
- enhanced team-member satisfaction with both their job and the leader
- reduced team-member stress and increased well-being
- enhanced quality of the services the team provide.

## Transactional and transformational leadership

These two styles of leadership (both discussed above) are not mutually exclusive. In transformational leadership, the power of the leader comes from creating understanding and trust and facilitating. While transformational leadership creates a high-performance culture within a team, elements of transactional leadership are required to ensure a clear focus on the achievement and measurement of results. This would suggest that an effective leader will be able to combine the two styles, so that targets, results and procedures are delivered by developing shared understanding and commitment.

If the benefits of transformational leadership are coupled with the benefits of transactional leadership, it is clear that this combination of leadership style would be particularly suitable for interprofessional team leaders. Table 4.2 illustrates features of an interprofessional team that make it suitable for a transformational/transactional style of leadership.

| Table 4.2 Interprofessional team features and leadership styles | |
|---|---|
| **Interprofessional team feature** | **Leadership style** |
| Day-to-day activities and tasks need to be achieved, for example, the care of a specific patient/client | Transactional |
| The team will need to work within the structures and boundaries of the organization | Transactional |
| The team is usually non-hierarchical, with the different professionals all working towards the same goals | Transformational |
| The team will have a long-term vision, which will be driven by government papers and policies | Transformational |
| The development needs of the individual team member are paramount, not only for the personal and professional development of the individual but also to the development of the team as a whole | Transformational |
| Team members are often working autonomously within an interprofessional team and therefore it is essential that they are empowered to control themselves and to manage their own problem solving | Transformational |

## Charismatic leadership (Conger and Kanungo, 1988, 1998)

The development of charismatic style of leadership is related to the type of environment that many organizations find themselves operating within in the 21st century. Today, many organizations, including the health and social care sectors, work in environments which are high risk, highly unpredictable and where there are rapid and often major changes taking place. These situations are characterized by high levels of anxiety and uncertainty that intensify processes of attribution, projection and transference and increase a perceived need for a charismatic leader. The charismatic leader is an image created by the followers, who use the leader as a 'screen' for their projections and attributions (Popper and Zakkai, 1994).

Conger and Kanungo (1998) identified five behaviours that are exhibited by charismatic leaders:

1 Can articulate a vision
2 Show sensitivity to members' needs
3 Show environmental sensitivity
4 Exhibit unconventional behaviour
5 Take personal risks

If these are the characteristics that a charismatic leader exhibits, what does a charismatic leader 'look' like? A charismatic leader uses their charm and personality to empower team members to believe in their own ability and to

**Internalize**
To accept or absorb an idea, belief, or opinion.

internalize the leader's vision before accepting it as their own. If this happens, it is likely that the leader will get their team members' respect. This style of leader will often deliver simple rather than complex visions.

A charismatic leader will show a great deal of interest in the team member that they are talking to at that moment, making the team member feel like they are, for that time, the most important person in the world. This type of leader is very perceptive and will be able to pick up on the moods and concerns of not only the individual team members but also the team as a whole. This enables the leader to focus their action and words to suit the situation at that moment in time.

A charismatic leader characteristically has a high level of self-belief, and will show enormous confidence in their team members. They are very persuasive and engender trust through taking personal risks in the name of their beliefs.

From the description thus far, it would appear that a charismatic leader possesses similar skills and attributes to those of a transformational leader. There is, however, one fundamental difference between the two styles of leadership and that is their basic focus. A transformational leader's focus is transforming the team and their team members, whereas a charismatic leader may not want to change anything, and may be more concerned with him or herself than anyone else.

There are some drawbacks to a charismatic leader:

- They have a tendency to dominate.
- They tend to prefer the 'big picture' to the detriment of the day-to-day operational detail of their vision.
- Their motives and strategies may not always be ethical.
- Team members become over reliant and dependent on their leader. If there is too much admiration the leader may feel that they are infallible. It is crucial that team members do not get swept along in a wave of enthusiasm created by their leader without stopping and questioning/re-examining the vision. Just because the leader believes something is right, it does not of course mean that it is right.
- They do not usually train and develop their successors and thus there is no natural successor if they leave the team or organization.
- They may be narcissistic and need power to cover their low self-esteem and possible lack of certain essential leadership skills. This potential lack of skills in a charismatic leader can be disastrous for the leader and their team members.

**Narcissistic**
An inflated sense of self-importance

## Authentic leadership

Authentic leadership is one of the newest areas of leadership research. In these challenging and turbulent times people feel insecure and apprehensive about what is going on around them and as a result they want leadership that they can trust and leaders who are honest and good (Avolio and Gardner, 2005). Authentic leadership is based on a clear focus on the positive role modeling of honesty, integrity, and high ethical standards in the development of leader–follower relationships (Wong and Cummings, 2009a).

George (2003) identified five dimensions of an authentic leader:

1 they understand their **purpose**
2 they have strong **values** about the right thing to do
3 they establish trusting **relationships** with others
4 they demonstrate **self discipline** and act on their values
5 they are passionate about their mission, that is, they act from their **heart**

For each of the five dimensions George (2003) identified five characteristics that individuals need to develop to become authentic leaders:

1 passion
2 behaviour
3 connectedness
4 consistency
5 compassion

A number of models have been developed to illustrate the process of authentic leadership (Gardner *et al.*, 2005; Ilies *et al.*, 2005; Luthans and Avolio, 2003). Walumbwa *et al.* (2008) identified four core components of authentic leadership: self-awareness, balanced information processing, internalized moral perspective (authentic behaviour) and relational transparency. Together these four components form the basis of authentic leadership (see Figure 4.3).

There are, however, other factors that influence authentic leadership (Northouse, 2010):

- positive psychological capacitates, for example, hope, optimism, resilience, confidence
- moral reasoning
- critical life events, for example, major events that shape your life and act as catalysts for change.

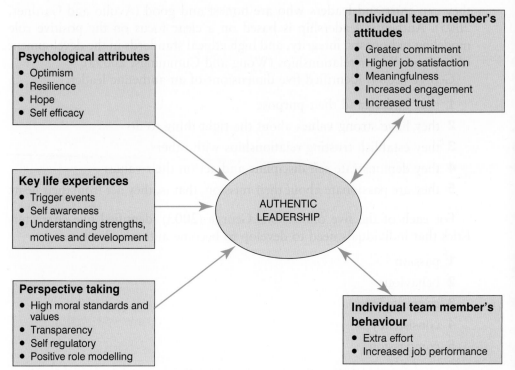

Figure 4.3   Key attributes of an authentic leader and the impact that these have on individual team members

In these unprecedented challenging times, there is a desire for higher standards of integrity, character and accountability of leaders, and the NHS is not exempt from this. It would, therefore, seem to be appropriate if we wish to develop healthier work environments for health and social care professionals that the NHS adopts authentic leadership. If the leader is supportive and there is trust in the management, staff will be more willing to raise concerns and put forward service improvement ideas and this will ultimately lead to a safer care environment and enhanced quality of care being provided to patients (Wong and Cummings, 2009b).

## What makes an effective team leader?

There is no doubt that the way in which a team is led will have a major impact upon the success or otherwise of the team. We are all able to identify a 'good' and a 'not so good' team leader, but what skills and behaviour does the team leader possess or not possess that leads us to make that decision?

## Reflective activity

Consider the skills, behaviour and qualities that you think make a good team leader.

### Leading a team

Maggie, a lead diagnostic radiographer is responsible for the day-to-day management of the CT Scanner. Her responsibilities include coordinating the workflow and directing a multidisciplinary team. The team includes at least one other senior radiographer with some skill and experience; a student radiographer; a trainee assistant practitioner; a radiologist who oversees the list and who is available for interventional procedures (biopsy/drainage), with a nurse as support. In addition, Maggie has to liaise closely with reception staff, secretarial staff (within the CT/medical imaging department), referring clinicians, ward staff and portering staff.

Maggie acts as a role model, providing strong clinical leadership underpinned by sound clinical practice, to promote a professional and smooth-running service (an effective and efficient service). She has the skills, knowledge, expertise and experience and furthermore the confidence, sense of responsibility, motivation and independence to deal with all situations within her department.

Maggie assesses the ability and willingness of the individuals within her team and adopts different leadership styles appropriate to the situation to encourage the members of her team to grow in all areas of their job.

Julie, a first-year student diagnostic radiographer, has just arrived as a new member of the team. As it is only her second day in the department, Maggie tells Julie what needs to be done. She gives very detailed instructions and supervises her closely to ensure that the tasks are being carried out correctly. For example, she asks Julie to help the patients change into a patient gown before their scans; collect the films from the processor; and assign them to the correct film packet ready for the radiologist to report.

Maggie also has a third-year diagnostic radiography student, Peter, in her team. Peter has experience of working in the CT scanning department and is keen to learn and willing to take responsibility. Maggie still gives him a lot of support and direction, but seeks Peter's involvement in the task, discussing the task with him, why it is necessary, how it can be best done.

James is the senior radiographer within Maggie's team. Maggie is able to allow him to take full responsibility for his work. She is, of course, there in the background to support James should that become necessary.

With reference to the case study:

- What type of leadership style do you think Maggie has adopted for Julie, Peter and James?
- What leadership skills do you think Maggie has?
- Are there any other skills that Maggie needs to effectively lead her multidisciplinary team?
- What do you think is Maggie's vision for her team?

In an attempt to draw together the qualities that an effective leader would require, the *NHS Leadership Framework* (NHS Leadership Academy, 2011) will be discussed. The Leadership Framework has been developed by the National Leadership Council and is for all staff working in health care, irrespective of discipline, role or function. The Framework is based on the concept that leadership is not restricted to those in a designated management position and that if we are going to transform services then there needs to be a shared responsibility to ensure success. Not everyone is necessarily a leader but everyone can contribute to the leadership process by using the behaviours described in the Leadership Framework.

The Leadership Framework consists of seven domains as can be seen in Figure 4.4. Within each domain there are four elements and each of these elements is further divided into four descriptors. It is the descriptors that describe the leadership behaviours, knowledge, skills or attitudes expected for each element.

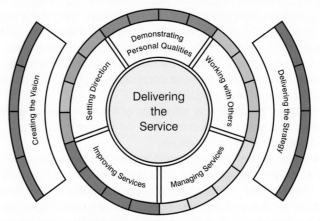

Figure 4.4   The seven domains of leadership
NHS Leadership Academy (2011) Available in the public domain from www.leadershipacademy.nhs.uk

As we have discussed, it is essential that health and social care professionals work together to ensure that effective and efficient care of a high quality is provided to patients. The domain 'Working with others' identifies the four elements that individuals must demonstrate effectiveness in.

1 Developing networks
2 Building and maintaining relationships
3 Encouraging contribution
4 Working within teams

If we look at the descriptors for one of these elements, 'Working within teams', we can see the four leadership behaviours which need to be demonstrated by the individual before they are considered a competent leader within this element. These are:

● Have a clear sense of their role, responsibilities and purpose within the team.
● Adopt a team approach, acknowledging and appreciating efforts, contributions and compromises.
● Recognize the common purpose of the team and respect team decisions.
● Willing to lead a team, involving the right people at the right time.

This Leadership Framework will underpin the new structures outlined by the coalition government (Department of Health, 2010a,b) and should ensure that the NHS is ready to deal with the many challenges that it faces in the future.

## EVIDENCE BASE

Go onto the website **www.nhsleadershipacademy.nhs.uk** and read about the Leadership Framework. The website provides full details of the Leadership Framework, including examples in practice for all seven domains and tools to help support you in using the Framework.

Spend time looking at all the descriptors for the four elements of the 'Working Together' domain. Reflect on how you might achieve competency within this domain.

## KEY POINTS

**Effective leaders:**

- possess qualities such as honesty, integrity, humility, courage, commitment, confidence, passion, determination and sensitivity
- make deliberate choices about how to tackle different situations and people
- do best when they adopt leadership styles that express their personality preferences and allow them to play to their strengths
- support the developmental needs of their individual team members
- are able to assess the competence levels of their team members and their commitment to completing tasks to achieve the required outcomes
- are able to balance the demands of the day-to-day tasks and team dynamics so that the needs of everyone involved in completing the task are taken into account
- have a vision and are able to motivate and inspire people to put the vision into practice
- want to make a real difference to people's health by delivering high-quality services and by developing the services provided by the team to patients and clients
- have a high level of self-awareness and know their own strengths and limitations.

## WHAT IS AN EXPERT?

As health and social care practitioners, we often remark that Sally or Julie or Imran are 'expert' practitioners and that we would be happy for that particular practitioner to care for us or a member of our family. But what makes an 'expert' practitioner, how do we know when we have seen one and why, in the context of interprofessional working, is it important to be able to define an expert practitioner? Using a case-study approach, we will discuss the issues raised by these questions.

## Health care professional

Two health care professionals were asked the same question related to their own profession: What is an 'expert'?

**Anja, a therapeutic radiographer, gave the following response:**

Knowledgeable, I think it's important to know things like side-effects, knowledge about a machine if you see something that's going a bit wrong, you can pick up minor faults before problems occur, knowledge on X-rays. I think an expert is organized, a team player, a good communicator so that they can communicate with the team and with patients as well, accurate, flexible and motivated. I also think that an expert has the confidence of experience, professionalism, technical ability, it's that judgement based upon experience, but still being able to treat that patient as an individual. It's knowing how far to go when and with what type of patient. For example, some patients like having your arm to lead them into the treatment room, while others might be offended by it, it's that judgement.

I think you can always tell your junior staff from senior staff in the way that they can deal with things. I think radiographers all have a lesson plan, perhaps a young-person lesson plan, a child lesson plan, an old-person lesson plan and even a patient-with-a-bladder-tumour lesson plan, because they've been there, it's an acceptable lesson plan and they're able to respond to those cues coming from the patient quickly. It's the adaptability, it's the expert element.

**Suresh, a mental-health nurse, gave this response:**

You want to know how an 'expert' mental-health nurse can be recognized? It's tempting to try and be funny but this is a serious question and not easy to answer. It is too obvious to say that this is a person who uses advanced knowledge, skill, education and experience in practice, although that is important. Alternatively, I could talk about their ability to establish an effective therapeutic alliance with the other. Um, no. Humanists would talk about the attributes of the complete person. Not terribly helpful.

I think the expert can be distinguished by the economic, skilful and smooth way in which they establish therapeutic alliances within their professional role. The expert mental-health nurse negotiates, with the client and themselves, about the purpose and activity of the relationship. They draw upon an extensive repertoire of skill and depth of experiential and theoretical knowledge. They don't always bring to conscious thought the whole of the decision-making process because some conclusions are less reasoned than intuitively known.

I believe that they operate in the most appropriate place on several scales:

Considered ..................................... spontaneous

Self-disclosing ....................................... private

Expressive ........................................ controlled

Also they avoid façades yet can function within required social roles, they have a healthy respect and liking for themselves that they extend to others. I also think that they have a childlike and warm sense of humour and engage with the other as person.

## Professional knowledge

As the concept of knowledge features prominently in Anja and Suresh's accounts, we will begin our exploration of expertise by discussing what is meant by professional knowledge.

The nature of professional knowledge is complex and it is difficult to define its exact nature. This should not, however, prevent us from attempting to tease out the essential meaning of professional knowledge. In this section, we will explore the various types of knowledge that make up the strands of professional knowledge.

Oakeshott (1962, cited in Eraut, 1994) makes a clear distinction between 'technical knowledge' and 'practical knowledge'. Technical knowledge, he suggests, is capable of written codification, that is, knowledge that can be articulated in the written form, for example in textbooks. Practical knowledge, on the other hand, is expressed only in practice and learned only through experience of practice. Practical knowledge has traditionally not been capable of written codification. Intuition and professional judgement are examples of practical knowledge.

**Propositional knowledge**
Knowledge based on facts and concepts

Patel *et al.* (1999) state that there are two basic types of knowledge: knowledge that can be verbalized, such as knowledge of facts and concepts; and knowledge that cannot be verbalized, such as intuition and knowledge of procedures. These two types of knowledge are referred to as propositional knowledge and non-propositional knowledge respectively.

Other authors have used different labels for these two types of knowledge, Ryle (1949) called them 'knowing that' and' knowing how', and Anderson (1983) referred to them as declarative knowledge and procedural knowledge (Table 4.3).

**Non-propositional knowledge**
Knowledge based on intuition and knowledge of procedures.

| Table 4.3 How authors have classified the two main types of knowledge | | |
|---|---|---|
| **Author** | **Knowledge that can be verbalized, e.g. facts** | **Knowledge which cannot be verbalized, e.g. intuition** |
| Ryle (1949) | 'Knowing that' | 'Knowing how' |
| Anderson (1983) | Declarative knowledge | Procedural knowledge |
| Oakeshott (cited in Eraut, 1994) | Technical knowledge | Practical knowledge |
| Patel *et al.* (1999) | Propositional knowledge | Non-propositional knowledge |

If we look at the 'Health care professional speaks' feature on page 80, we can see that both Anja and Suresh talk about these two different types of knowledge. Anja talks about experts needing knowledge of side-effects, X-rays and treatment machines. All of this knowledge can be found in a textbook and is, therefore, propositional knowledge.

Both Anja and Suresh refer to non-propositional knowledge. Suresh talks about experts not always bringing to conscious thought the whole of the decision-making process because some decisions are intuitively known. Anja mentions 'judgement based on experience' and practice being 'implied' rather than 'seen'. This suggests that Anja is distinguishing between the two types of knowledge, 'implied' referring to non-propositional knowledge and 'seen' referring to propositional knowledge.

**Personal knowledge**
Knowledge based on experience.

**Personal knowledge** is another strand of professional knowledge. Everyone acquires knowledge through experiences, either directly or vicariously, much of which does not have much apparent connection with learning. This type of knowledge has been referred to as personal knowledge (Kolb, 1984; Eraut, 1994; Fish, 1998). Many of the experiences we have are simply lived through unless the 'act of attention' halts the process and confers a meaning on the experience. When attention is focused more deeply upon an experience, it can be understood in a meaningful way. One important way in which health and social care practitioners 'halt' this process, and thus give meaning to their experiences, is by reflecting on their practice.

However, personal knowledge is not created in a vacuum but is constructed through interaction with the social, political, economical and cultural context in which the experience occurs. This latter knowledge is referred to as social knowledge, which Kolb defines as:

**Social knowledge**
Knowledge constructed from interaction with the social, political, economical and cultural context in which the experience occurs.

> *independent, socially and culturally transmitted networks of words, symbols and images based solely on comprehension*
>
> *Kolb (1984, p. 105)*

Personal knowledge and social knowledge can be seen as complementary, with an individual's development being the product of the transaction between personal experience and the system of social knowledge interacted with.

Vygotsky's (1978) work emphasizes the societal context of an individual's cognitive development. Central to his theory is the concept of the 'zone of proximal development', in which a novice's development occurs through participation in activities slightly beyond their competence with the assistance of more skilled practitioners. Learning takes place in the zone of proximal development via interactions between an individual's personal knowledge system and the society within which the learning is taking place.

For the purposes of description, it may be easy to separate out the different types of knowledge: propositional knowledge; non-propositional knowledge; personal knowledge; social knowledge, but during practice the different types of knowledge are inextricably linked. As Williams succinctly states:

> *During professional action, knowledge becomes a dynamic integrated 'whole' which is shaped and adapted to fit each situation which is encountered.*
>
> *Williams (1998, p. 29)*

Professional knowledge is not a discrete entity and undoubtedly the development of professional knowledge is affected by the social, cultural, historical, attitudinal, psychological and behavioural context that the individual is operating within. However, making practical knowledge more explicit and thus accessible for codification, criticism and dissemination would help to enhance understanding of the nature of expertise, in the health and social care professions. Also when working within an interprofessional team, it is important that practitioners are able to make their practical knowledge accessible to others in the team. In this way, practitioners will be able to appreciate, for example, how and why individual members of the team arrive at specific decisions or problem-solve in a particular way. An important part of this process is to be able to define what makes an 'expert' practitioner.

## KEY POINTS

**The strands of professional knowledge are:**

- propositional knowledge
- non-propositional knowledge
- personal knowledge
- social knowledge

## Experience and expertise

If we look back again at the 'Health care professional speaks' feature on page 80 we can see that Anja and Suresh have used the word 'experience' to describe an important characteristic of an expert practitioner in their field of practice. But what does 'experience' actually mean and how does it forward an understanding of what an expert practitioner is? As the concept of experience features prominently in Anja and Suresh's accounts and also within the literature on expertise, it would suggest that an understanding of the nature of experience would be useful when defining an expert. The definition of 'experience' is often taken for granted, yet there appears to be no agreement within the literature as to what constitutes an experience. A dictionary definition of 'experience' does not encapsulate the holistic nature of experience but breaks it into its component parts, for example 'the knowledge or skill acquired by a period of practical experience of something', 'practical contact with and observation of facts or events', 'an event or occurrence which leaves an impression on someone' (*Oxford Dictionaries*, 2012). Oakeshott (1933, cited in Boud *et al.*, 1993, p. 9) sees experience as having two elements, 'experiencing' and 'what is experienced', and that these two elements compose a single whole.

Kolb (1984, p. 35) makes the following comments about experience.

> *The transactional relationship between the person and the environment ... symbolized in the dual meanings of the term experience – one subjective and personal referring to the person's internal state ... and the other objective and environmental.*

Boud *et al.* (1993, p. 9) characterize experience as having 'within it judgement, thought and connectedness with other experience – it is not isolated'. This definition suggests that experience is a meaningful encounter.

Ericsson (1996, p. 9) makes reference to a 'ten-year rule of preparation' before an individual becomes an expert in their chosen domain. To support this rule, Ericsson (1996) cites a number of studies: Simon and Chase (1973), who suggested that no one became a grand master in chess in fewer than nine to ten years, and Patel *et al.* (1996) who speak of the necessity of ten years' preparation before a doctor can call themselves an expert.

Clearly, experience is important for the achievement of expertise, but it is the nature of this accrued experience that will determine whether an individual will become an expert. The simple accumulation of practice is not sufficient; if you endlessly repeat the same exercise, you will not develop into an expert. Time must be accompanied by the chance to accumulate a varied set of meaningful experiences.

## Models for developing expertise

Various models for developing expertise can be found within the literature. This section will describe two of these models:

1 The Dreyfus model of skill acquisition (Dreyfus and Dreyfus, 1986).
2 The cognitive continuum theory (Hammond, 1980).

It is important to discuss these models of expertise as they provide an insight into the way in which an expert practitioner develops. These models highlight that an interprofessional team will have practitioners not only from different professions but also at different stages of their development, in other words, practitioners will have more or less expertise in their field than other practitioners within their team.

### Dreyfus and Dreyfus (1986) model of skill acquisition

This model has as its key contextual feature, experience. Hubert Dreyfus, a philosopher, and Stuart Dreyfus, an operations researcher, describe a five-stage model for the development of expertise. An individual must go through each stage to become an expert in their domain, the five stages being novice, advanced beginner, competent, proficient and expert. The movement from novice to expert relies upon the practitioner accumulating situated practical experience and is characterized by the use of intuitive thinking as opposed to analytical thinking and the ability of the practitioner to see a situation as a whole rather than just its individual parts.

As already stated, experience is the key feature of this model. It is the practitioner's experience with a particular task that determines the cognitive mode selected; for example, a novice is by definition unfamiliar with the task and will adopt an analytic, step-by-step approach. As the novice gains more experience and becomes an advanced beginner, a competent practitioner and then a proficient practitioner, the balance between analytical and intuitive thinking alters so that by the time a practitioner becomes an expert all decisions pertaining to a particular task are carried out intuitively. Dreyfus and Dreyfus (1986, p. 30–31) state:

> " An expert generally knows what to do based on mature and practical understanding … an expert's skill has become so much part of him that he need be no more aware of it than he is of his own body … when things are proceeding normally experts don't solve problems and don't make decisions; they do what normally works.

A criticism of the Dreyfus and Dreyfus model is the difficulty in applying the five levels of expertise. Practitioners rarely perform at the same level on all tasks in a domain. A therapeutic radiographer may perform at the level of expert when performing tasks that they frequently encounter, for example, discussing with patients the acute side-effects that may result from the radiotherapy treatment they are about to receive. Whereas they may perform at the level of proficiency for tasks they encounter less frequently, for example. 'setting up' patients suffering from cancer of the head and neck region, localizing and planning radiotherapy treatments. For tasks that are relatively unfamiliar, for example, the application of specialized techniques, the therapeutic radiographer would perform at the level of competence. So it would be a mistake to label a particular therapeutic radiographer as an expert and expect them to perform consistently at that level in all tasks in the domain of therapeutic radiography. A more accurate definition of an expert would be an individual who is capable of handling a wide range of tasks intuitively, compared to an individual with less experience.

## EVIDENCE BASE

Go onto the website **http://www.gp-training.net/training/educational_theory/adult_learning/ skill.htm** and read about the Dreyfus and Dreyfus (1986) model of skill acquisition. This website provides descriptors for each of the five levels of skill acquisition.

Another criticism of the Dreyfus and Dreyfus model is that it claims that novices only think analytically and that experts only think intuitively.

Dreyfus and Dreyfus (1986) argue that, because novices are unfamiliar with the task, they have to take an analytical approach. But you could argue that the unfamiliarity of the task induces intuition because the novice has not learnt any analytic principles for organizing their thinking about the situation, and thus has to rely on the intuitive method for integrating information (Hamm, 1999).

The Dreyfus and Dreyfus model fails, therefore, to recognize the crucial role that the task plays in influencing the individual to select the appropriate cognitive mode.

### Cognitive continuum theory (Hammond, 1980)

This model of expertise, developed by the psychologist Kenneth Hammond, recognizes the important role that the task plays in the development of expertise. This theory has three elements: a cognitive continuum, a task continuum and a range of modes of practice. Unlike the Dreyfus and Dreyfus model, which speaks of two pure types of cognition, analytical for novices and intuitive for experts, Hammond (1980) believes that analytical and intuitive thinking should be placed on the poles of a continuum. This is because most thinking is neither purely analytical nor purely intuitive but lies somewhere in between.

The cognitive continuum is of little value to the practitioner if there is no indication as to which kind of thinking to use in various situations. Therefore, to enable the practitioner to convert the idea of the cognitive continuum into guidance about how to think, the task becomes important. The task continuum ranges from analysis-inducing to intuition-inducing and the position that a task occupies on the continuum depends on the type of task, for example the complexity of the task, the ambiguity of the task content and the form of task presentation (Hamm, 1999). Thus, the cognitive continuum theory recognizes that it is possible for an expert to think analytically in one situation and intuitively in another depending on the type of task. Dreyfus and Dreyfus claim, conversely, that being an expert means that the individual must take an intuitive approach to all tasks within their domain.

This last point raises another question. If an individual uses intuitive cognition to make decisions, will a greater degree of accuracy be achieved than if analytical cognition is used? Hammond (1980) argues that it is not the mode of cognition that affects the accuracy of a decision, but whether the appropriate mode of cognition has been selected for the task. For example, if the conditions of a task suggest that an analytical approach should be adopted but the individual tries to use an intuitive approach, then errors can occur. Conversely, if the task suggests that an intuitive approach should be adopted and the individual tries to use an analytic approach, then poor performance may result (Hamm, 1999). The evidence suggests that experts perform by way of a variety of cognitive modes, depending on the task, and that this variation is good because an expert's intuition is not infallible in all situations.

Neither the Dreyfus and Dreyfus model nor the cognitive continuum theory has attempted to explain how an individual becomes an expert, only that experience, type of task and modes of cognition have a role in the development of an expert.

## Knowledge and expertise

In this section we consider the relationship between knowledge and expertise. Research into expertise has focused on differences between individuals varying in levels of expertise, in terms of memory, reasoning strategies and the role of domain-specific knowledge.

Anja and Suresh, as already discussed in the 'Health care professional speaks' feature on page 80, both make reference to knowledge and expertise in their practice. It may appear to be stating the obvious that there is a link between knowledge base and expertise. However, what is important is not only having an extensive body of knowledge but that the knowledge is organized in such a way that it is accessible and useable.

The way in which knowledge is represented in memory has a not insignificant role to play in the differences observed in problem solving by experts and novices. Research has indicated that experts appear to have the following characteristics: experts use forward reasoning to problem solve, whereas novices try to solve problems in a backward way (Simon and Simon, 1978); experts take a more direct route to problem solving than novices (Patel *et al.*, 1994) and that experts problem solve faster and more economically than novices (Chi *et al.*, 1988; Schmidt *et al.*, 1990).

The notion of 'schemes of experience' (Schutz, 1967), frames (Minsky, 1977), scripts (Schank and Abelson, 1977), templates (Boreham, 1988) and illness scripts (Schmidt *et al.*, 1990) will be used to explore these differences in problem solving between novices and experts. Although all of these schemata are subtly different, they all have the same underlying principle, that is, they:

> ❝❝ *attempt to describe how acquired knowledge is organized and represented and how such cognitive structures facilitate the use of knowledge in particular ways.*
>
> *Glaser (1984, p. 100)*

Schmidt *et al.*'s (1990) four-stage model of medical expertise recognizes that personal experience as well as propositional knowledge has an important role in the development of what Schmidt *et al.* refer to as 'illness scripts', which are developed during stage three of this model. The clinical experience of the medical practitioner becomes increasingly important during stage three, when illness scripts are being developed, and stage four, when memories of previous patients are being maintained. Stage one is solely concerned with the gaining of knowledge and its development into a network with links made between related pieces of information. It is stage two that is particularly important in the context of this discussion. Stage two involves the transformation of the networks developed by medical students in stage one into abridged networks using high-level causal models, with information about signs and symptoms being subsumed under 'diagnostic labels'. Thus, the medical student is now able to represent a disease in their memory, for example, bowel cancer, as opposed to seeing the disease as its individual signs and symptoms, for example, diarrhoea, rectal bleeding, pain and so on. As the medical student has had more practical experience, it is possible for them to select only the most critical information and to disregard the irrelevant information to solve a problem.

The idea that performance improves when the individual has access to multiple experiences/stories is important in relation to an expert's superior problem-solving capacities. During stage three of Schmidt *et al.*'s model, 'illness scripts' are developed and these illness scripts provide the medical practitioner with multiple experiences/stories, which they can use when making medical diagnoses. The development of illness scripts is dependent on accumulated experience of working with patients and thus this also supports the generally accepted view that substantial experience is required for expert performance. During stage four, the medical practitioner stores memories of previous patients and, therefore, during stages three and four medical practitioners accumulate numerous rich schemata which they can draw upon to problem solve.

Schemata such as those developed by Schmidt *et al.*'s model go some way to explaining why experts take a more direct route to problem solving compared to novices. The more experienced a practitioner is, the greater the number of schemata they will have accumulated and the more able they will be to use forward reasoning as a problem-solving strategy. For example, if a therapeutic radiographer has seen the same physical and psychological effects arising from treating a patient with a tumour of the pelvic region many times, for example, diarrhoea, nausea and vomiting, anxiety, loss of self-esteem and so on, then they are more likely to recognize important cues that will lead more directly to a solution the next time this situation is encountered.

Anja's case study (see 'Health care professional speaks' feature on page 80) illustrates this point by reference to the range of 'lesson plans' that therapeutic radiographers have developed through experience. The 'lesson plans' which Anja refers to appear to be serving the same function as 'illness scripts'.

As schema theory assumes that there are schemata for recurrent situations, then one of the major functions of these schemata will be to construct interpretations of situations, such as those just described. A novice therapeutic radiographer, who by definition will have less accumulated knowledge and therefore fewer schemata to draw upon, will have to think through the problem more explicitly and make more inferences before arriving at a correct solution to the problem.

**Schemata**
Frameworks for organising ideas about the world or new information.

In conclusion, researchers have taken two different approaches to defining an expert. Models of expertise have been developed, for example, the model of skill acquisition (Dreyfus and Dreyfus, 1986), the four-stage model of clinical expertise (Schmidt *et al.*, 1990) and the cognitive continuum theory (Hammond, 1980). These models, however, do not explain how an individual becomes an expert. The second approach appears to address the 'how' by identifying characteristics of an expert performance and explaining the cognitive processes involved. However, it would appear that there is no single 'expert way' to perform all tasks. Dorner and Scholkopf's (1991) general characterization of expert performance is most apt, 'An expert is someone capable of doing the right thing at the right time'.

## KEY POINTS

The key characteristics of an expert:

- experts are knowledgeable and have a deep level of propositional knowledge and a large volume of non-propositional knowledge
- experts are reflective practitioners
- experts are highly motivated and internally driven
- experts excel mainly in their own domain
- experts are faster at performing the skills in their domain
- experts are fast at solving problems and make few errors
- experts value the participation of relevant others in the decision-making process
- experts are patient centred
- experts share their expertise to help develop expertise in others.

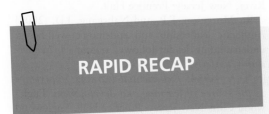

## RAPID RECAP

Check your progress so far by working through each of the following questions.

1 What are the main types of leadership style?

2 What leadership styles are usually adopted by an interprofessional team leader?

3 What skills and qualities does an effective team leader possess?

4 What are the strands of professional knowledge?

5 List five of the key characteristics of an expert.

If you have difficulty with more than one of the questions, read through the section again to refresh your understanding before moving on.

# REFERENCES

Anderson, J.R. (1983) *The architecture of cognition*. Cambridge, MA: Harvard University Press.

Avolio, B.J. and Bass, B.M. (1988) Transformational leadership, charisma, and beyond. In *Emerging leadership* (eds. Hunt, J.G., Baglia, B.R., Dachler, H.P. and Scriescheim, C.A.). Lexington, MA: Lexington Books, pp. 29–50.

Avolio, B.J. and Gardner, W.L. (2005) Authentic leader-ship development: getting to the root of positive forms of leadership. *The Leadership Quarterly* **16**: 315–338.

Barr, J. and Dowding, L. (2012) *Leadership in health care*, 2nd ed. London: Sage Publications.

Bass, B.M. (1985) *Leadership performance beyond expectations*. New York: The Free Press.

Bass, B.M. and Avolio, B.J. (1994) *Improving effectiveness through transformational leadership*. Thousand Oaks, CA: Sage Publications.

Boreham, N.C. (1988) Models of diagnosis and their implications for adult professional education. In *Studies in the Education of Adults*, **20**: 95–108.

Boud, D., Cohen, R. and Walker, D. (1993) *Using experience for learning*. Milton Keynes: Open University Press.

Burns, J.M. (1978) *Leadership*. New York: Harper & Row.

Chi, M.T.H., Glaser, R. and Farr, M. (1988) *The nature of expertise*. Erlbaum, NJ Hillsdale, NJ.

Cohen, G. (2009) Defining leadership. *Leadership excellence*. **26**(8): 16–17.

Conger, J.A. and Kanungo, R. (1988) *Charismatic leadership: the elusive factor in organizational effectiveness*. San Francisco, CA: Jossey-Bass Publishers.

Conger, J.A. and Kanungo, R. (1998) *Charismatic leadership in organizations*. Thousand Oaks: Sage Publications, CA.

Department of Health (2010a) *Equity and excellence: liberating the NHS*. London: HMSO.

Department of Health (2010b) *A vision for adult social care: capable communities and active citizens*. London: HMSO.

Dorner, D. and Scholkopf, J. (1991) Controlling complex systems; or, expertise as 'Grandmother's know-how'. In *Toward a general theory of expertise* (eds. Ericsson, K.A. and Smith, J.). Cambridge: Cambridge University Press, pp. 218–239.

Dreyfus, H.L. and Dreyfus, S.E. (1986) *Mind over machine: the power of human intuition and expertise in the era of the computer*. New York: The Free Press.

Eraut, M. (1994) *Developing professional knowledge and competence*. London: Falmer Press.

Ericsson, K.A. (1996) The acquisition of expert performance: an introduction to some of the issues. In *The road to excellence: the acquisition of expert performance in the arts and sciences, sports and games* (ed. Ericsson, K.A.). Hillsdale, NJ Lawrence Erlbaum Associates, pp. 1–50.

Fish, D. (1998) *Appreciating practice in the caring professions: re-focusing professional development and practitioner research*. Oxford: Butterworth-Heinemann.

Gardner, W.L., Avolio, B.J., Luthans, F., May, D.R. and Walumba, F. (2005) 'Can you see the real me?' A self-based model of authentic leader and follower development. *The Leadership Quarterly*. **16**: 343–372.

George, B. (2003) *Authentic leadership: rediscovering the secrets to creating lasting value*. San Francisco, CA: Jossey-Bass.

Glaser, R. (1984) The role of knowledge. *American Psychologist*, **79**(2): 93–104.

Hamm, R.M. (1999) Clinical expertise and the cognitive continuum. In *Professional judgement: a reader in clinical decision making* (eds. Dowie, J. and Elstein, A.). Cambridge: The Open University Press, pp. 78–105.

Hammond, K. (1980) *Human judgement and decision making*. New York: Hemisphere.

Hersey, P. and Blanchard, K.H. (1977) *The management of organizational behaviour*. Upper Saddle River, New Jersey: Prentice Hall.

Ilies, R., Morgeson, F.P. and Nahrgang, J.D. (2005) Authentic leadership and eudemonic well-being: understanding leader-follower outcomes. *Leadership Quarterly*,**16**: 373–394.

Kolb, D.A. (1984) *Experiential learning: experience as the source of learning and development*. Englewood Cliffs New Jersey: Prentice Hall, Englewood Cliffs.

Kirkpatrick, S.A. and Locke, E.A. (1991) Leadership: do traits matter? *The Executive*. **5**: 48–60.

Luthans, F. and Avolio, B.J. (2003) Authentic leadership development. In *Positive organizational scholarship* (eds. Cameron, K.S., Dutton, J.E and Quinn, R.E.) San Fransico: Berrett-Koehler, pp. 241–258.

Mann, R.D. (1959) A review of the relationship between personality and performance in small groups. *Psychological Bulletin*. **56**: 241–270.

Minsky, M. (1977) Frame-system Theory. In *Thinking: readings in cognitive science* (eds. Johnson-Laird,

P.N. and Watson, P.C.). Cambridge: Cambridge University Press, pp. 355–367.

National Health Service Leadership Academy (2011) The leadership framework. Available from: **www.leadershipacademy.nhs.uk**. Accessed June 2012.

Northouse, P.G. (2010) *Leadership: theory and practice,* 5th edition. London: Sage Publications.

Oxford Dictionaries [online] (2012) Available at **http://oxforddictionaries.com**.

Patel, V.L., Arocha, J.F. and Kaufman, D.R. (1994) Diagnostic reasoning and expertise. *The Psychology of Learning and Motivation: Advances in Research Theory.* 31: 137–252.

Patel, V.L., Arocha, J.F. and Kaufman, D.R. (1999) Expertise and tacit knowledge in medicine. In *Tacit knowledge in professional practice* (Sternberg, R.J. and Horvath, J.A.). Hillsdale, NJ: Lawrence Erlbaum Associates, pp. 75–99.

Patel, V.L., Kaufmann, D.R. and Magder, S.A. (1996) The acquisition of medical expertise in complex dynamic environments. In *The road to excellence: The acquisition of expert performance in the arts and sciences, sports and games* (ed. Ericsson, K.A.). Hillsdale, NJ: Lawrence Erlbaum Associates, pp. 1–50.

Popper, M. and Zakkai, E. (1994) Transactional, charismatic and transformational leadership: conditions conducive to their predominance. *Leadership & Organization Development Journal,* 15(6): 3–7.

Ryle, G. (1949) *The concept of mind.* London: Penguin.

Schank, R. and Abelson, R.P. (1977) Scripts, plans and knowledge. In *Thinking: readings in cognitive science* (eds. Johnson-Laird, P.N. and Wanson, P.C.). Cambridge: Cambridge University Press, pp. 421–432.

Schmidt, H.G., Norman, G.R. and Boshuizen, H. (1990) A cognitive perspective on medical expertise: theory and implications. In *Academic Medicine,* 65(10): 611–621.

Schutz, A. (1967) *The phenomenology of the social world.* Evanston, IL: North Western University Press.

Simon, D.P. and Simon, H.A. (1978) Individual differences in solving physics problems. In *Children's thinking: what develops?* (ed. Siegler, R.S.). Hillsdale, NJ: Lawrence Erlbaum Associates, pp. 325–348.

Simon, H.A. and Chase, W.G. (1973) Skill in chess. *American Scientist,* 61: 394–403.

Stogdhill, R.M. (1974) *Handbook of leadership: a survey of the literature.* New York: Free Press.

Vroom, V.H. and Jago, A.G. (2007) The role of situation in leadership. *American Psychologist.* 62(1): 17–24.

Vygotsky, L.S. (1978) *Mind in society. The development of higher psychological processes.* Cambridge, MA: Harvard University Press.

Walumbwa, F., Avolio, B., Gardner, W., Wernsing, T. and Peterson, S. (2008) Authentic leadership: development and validation of a theory based measure. *Journal of Management.* 34(1): 89–126.

Williams, P. (1998) Using Theories of professional knowledge and reflective practice to influence educational change. *Medical Teacher,* 20(1): 28–34.

Wong, C.A. and Cummings, G.G. (2009a) The influence of authentic leadership behaviours on trust and work outcomes of health care staff. *Journal of Leadership Studies.* 3(2): 6–23.

Wong, C.A. and Cummings, G.G. (2009b) Authentic leadership: a new theory for nursing or back to basics? *Journal of Health Organization and Management.* 23(5): 522–538.

Zaccaro, S.J., Kemp, C., and Bader, P. (2004) Leader traits and attributes. In *The Nature of Leadership* (eds Antonakis, J., Cianciolo, A.T. and Sternburg, R.J.). Thousand Oaks, CA: Sage, pp. 101–124.

# CHAPTER 5

# COMMUNICATING WITH EACH OTHER

## LEARNING OBJECTIVES

*By the end of this chapter you should be able to:*

- Discuss the fundamental communication skills needed to facilitate effective relationships with patients, carers and health care professionals

- Identify the methods of communication that enhance effective interprofessional working

- Discuss the barriers to effective communication.

## INTRODUCTION

Effective communication is considered to be essential for effective interprofessional working and the consequent delivery of quality health and social care to patients. Communication covers a wide range of interactions including interpersonal communication, communication technology and mass communication. It also takes many forms: from brief informal conversations between professionals, to formal meetings, for example, multidisciplinary team meetings; from ward rounds through to formalized written documents between professionals, for example. patients records or case notes. Whether the type of communication is verbal or written the purpose is always the same, that is, the sharing of information.

All too often we have seen the tragic deaths that have occurred from a breakdown in communication within different parts of the NHS and between the NHS and other care providers such as social services. Deaths such as that of Baby Peter (see *Serious Case Review*, LSCB Haringey, 2009), Victoria Climbié (see report, Secretary of State for Health, 2003) and the children undergoing heart surgery at Bristol Royal Infirmary (see report, Secretary of State for Health, 2001). Failures in mental health care, for example the death of Father Paul Bennett who was killed by Geraint Evans, paranoid schizophrenic (Health care Inspectorate Wales, 2009) and the death of a ten-day-old baby boy by his mother, Katy Norris, who was suffering from severe post-natal depression (Torbay Safeguarding Children Board, *Serious Case Review*, 2010). The reports into these deaths all made recommendations related to the communication skills of health and social care professionals (see Box 5.1, 5.2 and 5.3).

There can be no doubt, as the recommendations following these tragic deaths so vividly illustrate, about the crucial role that effective communication has in the delivery of effective patient and client care.

Since 2002 (Department of Health, 2000) it has been a pre-condition of qualification to deliver patient care in the NHS that an individual has demonstrated competence in communication with patients. The following skills were identified (Department of Health 2003a) as being necessary for students to possess at the point of registration. Students should:

- Be able to identify the communication skills required in practice to improve patient-care management and patient satisfaction with their care
- Have the ability to communicate effectively with fellow professionals and other health care staff
- Have the ability to recognize the level of their communication skills and limitations in specialist practice and be committed to personal development in these areas through post-registration and continuing professional development opportunities throughout their careers.

The deaths of baby Peter, Victoria Climbié, the children undergoing heart surgery at Bristol, Leo Norris, Father Paul Bennett and many high profile deaths of children and adults serve to further reinforce the requirement for health and social care professionals to possess appropriate competencies in communication skills.

## BOX 5.1

**The report (Secretary of State for Health, 2001) into the deaths of children from heart surgery at Bristol Royal Infirmary**

This had among its recommendations the following:

**Recommendation 59**

Education in communication skills must be an essential part of the education of all health care professionals. Communication skills include the ability to engage with patients on an emotional level, to listen, to assess how much information a patient wants to know and to convey information with clarity and sympathy.

**Recommendation 60**

Communication skills must also include the ability to engage with and respect the views of fellow health care professionals.

# BOX 5.2

**The report into the death of Victoria Climbié (Secretary of State for Health, 2003)**

This had a significant number of recommendations that focused on written communication including the following:

**Recommendation 12**

Front-line staff in each of the agencies which regularly come into contact with families with children must ensure that with each new contact, basic information about the child is recorded. This must include the child's name, address, age, the name of the child's primary carer, the child's GP and the name of the child's school if the child is of school age.

**Recommendation 37**

The training of social workers must equip them with the confidence to question the opinion of professionals in other agencies when conducting their own assessment of the needs of the child.

**Recommendation 38**

Directors of social services must ensure that the transfer of responsibility of a case between local authority social services departments is always recorded on the case file of each authority and is confirmed in writing by the authority to which responsibility for the case has been transferred.

**Recommendation 68**

When concerns about deliberate harm of a child have been raised, doctors must ensure that comprehensive and contemporaneous notes are made of these concerns.

Other recommendations within the report into the death of Victoria Climbié (Secretary of State for Health, 2003) focused on the sharing and accessing of information between agencies.

# BOX 5.3

**The report into the death of Father Paul Bennett (Health care Inspectorate Wales, 2009)**

This had a significant number of recommendations for various agencies that focused on written and verbal communication including the following:

**Accident and Emergency (A&E)**
**Recommendation 3.1a**

Communication between A&E department, other departments and GPs is subject to formal arrangements, including immediate telephone contact when necessary, formal written reports and routine auditing.

**Community mental health services**
**Recommendation 3.2e**

Communication with other agencies is timely and effective and that any follow up is carried out fully and comprehensively.

**Recommendation 3.2f**

All agencies need to meet together in order to discuss how to handle complex cases and develop a comprehensive care pathway.

**The Health Board and Local Authorities**
**Recommendation 3.3g**

Records are accurately documented and reviewed in order to aid with spotting any patterns which may emerge in relation to the risk assessment process.

**Recommendation 3.3h**

Record management arrangements are robust and routinely audited and that records are kept secure are all times.

We will begin this chapter by exploring the different methods of communication that are used in the health and social care sector to enhance interprofessional working and the quality of care delivered to patients and clients. Next, we will discuss the various types of team communication and enabling technologies. Finally, we will consider the barriers to communicating effectively within an interprofessional working environment and how these barriers might be overcome.

## METHODS OF COMMUNICATION

In health and social care, the word 'communication' covers a wide range of interactions, which can broadly be classified into two types: verbal communication and written communication.

### Verbal communication

It is important to remember that, when we communicate verbally, it is not just the words and phrases of the spoken language that convey our message but also our non-verbal actions. In fact usually more information is gained from non-verbal communication than from the words that someone is actually saying. It has been found that people's attitudes and feelings are communicated 55 per cent by the body, 38 per cent by the voice and only 7 per cent by spoken words (Chapman, 2012).

Being able to communicate effectively within the fields of health and social care is paramount as it can mean the difference between life and death. A vital partnership exists between health and social care professionals themselves, and between health and social care professionals and their patients that can be either negatively or positively affected by interprofessional communication. It is, therefore, crucial that all health and social care professionals continuously enhance their communication skills to enable them to work effectively within an interprofessional team.

Verbal communication is the primary way in which health and social care professionals transmit information about a patient's care and treatment. To enhance interprofessional working, health and social care professionals use both formal and informal, direct (face-to-face) verbal communication strategies. Formal strategies include team meetings, ward rounds, child protection strategy meetings, children in need planning meetings and multidisciplinary team meetings. Informal communication strategies tend to be opportunistic interactions including 'catching' other professionals in the hospital corridors; verbal updates between professionals to communicate any new decisions on patient management.

Verbal communication is generally much less structured and less consistent than written communication. When information is communicated verbally there are few, if any, guidelines to ensure the accuracy and completeness of the information being exchanged. There is, therefore, a risk that valuable information might be misinterpreted or lost, for example, staff may forget some of the information so that an incomplete message is passed on, or staff may forget to pass the message on. If information is lost, misinterpreted or is incomplete, a breakdown of communication will result, with consequent effects on patient care. It is, therefore, essential that as health and social care professionals you are aware of the barriers to effective verbal communication and how these might be overcome.

## Reflective activity

This exercise will help you think about the purpose and outcome of communication that you have been involved in whilst in practice.

Keep a communication diary for a day whilst in your practice placement, writing down everybody you spoke to in a 24-hour period.

- List who are the people that you interacted with.

- For each person you have listed identify the purpose of the communication and what the outcome was.

- Critically reflect and analyse three of these interactions and think whether the desired outcome was achieved.

- For each of the interactions you have identified think about how you could enhance your communication skills in the future.

## Reflective activity

Whilst the words that we use to communicate are important it is our non-verbal communication skills that are likely to more dominant in any conversation that we have with a patient or another health or social care professional. The main aspects of non-verbal communication are body language; proximity; body orientation; posture; touch; gestures; facial expression; and eye contact.

This exercise will help you think about the impact that non-verbal communication may have on the information that you are conveying to a patient. Think about two different scenarios when you have been involved in communicating with a patient. For each scenario think about the non-verbal messages that you were conveying by considering the following questions:

- How were you dressed and what appearance did you present to the patient?

- How was the room arranged?

- Did you manage the space between you and the patient appropriately?

- What was your posture like?

- Did you fidget?

- What did your facial expressions and gestures convey?

- What were your eyes doing during the conversation?

- Did you have any body contact with the patient?

Health and social care professionals also use indirect verbal communication which is usually used as a formal communication strategy. Indirect verbal communication is any verbal communication that is not face to face, for example, via the telephone, video conferencing, teleconferencing, the answer phone, SMS text messaging.

## EVIDENCE BASE

SMS text messaging is used in a number of ways in the UK to deliver health care, including as a reminder service, for providing test results, for providing specialist information, and wellness and motivation programmes, for example, smoking cessation.

Go to the website **http://www.institute.nhs.uk/building_capability/technology_and_ product_innovation/text_messaging.html**

This site provides useful information on text messaging and gives links to examples where text messaging is actually being used in health care settings.

## Written communication

There are a variety of different types of written communication that health and social care professionals use to communicate information, including: letters, fax, notice boards, e-mails, newsletters, reports, minutes from meetings, incident/accident forms. In addition to these general types of written communication, there are those that are specific to the health and social care setting including: prescriptions, death certificates, patient records, investigation request cards, medicine/drug charts, vital-signs charts.

## Reflective activity

This activity will help you to think about the range of written communication methods that you come across in your practice.

1 List the types of written communication that you use in your practice area.

2 Identify the advantages and disadvantages of the types of written communication that you have identified.

3 Take one of the types of written communication you have identified and consider how you might make it more effective to enhance the quality of care provided to the patient.

## EVIDENCE BASE

E-mail communication is now being used in the delivery of health care in the UK.

Read the following three articles to find out more about how e-mail communication and the Internet is being used to improve health and social care outcomes.

- Sheaves, B., Jones, R., Williamson, G. and Chauhan, R. (2011) Phase I pilot of e-mail support for people with long term conditions using the Internet. *BMC Medical Informatics and Decision Making.***11**:20. This article can be accessed from **http://www.biomedcentral.com/1472-6947/11/20**.

- Dean, A. (2008) Communicating with patients using email and the internet. *Nursing Times.net.***104**:7. This article can be accessed from **http://www.nursingtimes.net/nursing-practice-clinical-research/communicating-with-patients-using-email-and-the-internet/755620.article**.

- Dodsworth, J., Bailey, S., Schofield, G., Cooper, N., Fleming, P. and Young, J. (2012) Internet technology: An empowering or alienating tool for communication between foster-carers and social worker? *British Journal of Social Work.* doi:10.1093/bjsw/bcs007

Go to the website **http://www.institute.nhs.uk/building_capability/technology_and_product_innovation/email.html**

This site provides useful information on email and provides links to examples where text messaging is being used in health care settings.

Health and social care organizations have developed guidelines and procedures to address certain methods of written communication, such as which parts of the patient's case record or forms should be completed at each stage of the patient's journey to and through a team. For example, when a patient is referred for treatment, a referral form will be completed; when a patient is admitted to a ward a nursing assessment sheet will be completed; during a patient's stay in hospital a nursing care plan, vital-signs chart and a drug chart will be completed; and when a patient is discharged from the ward, a discharge plan will be completed.

Structured documents/forms designed specifically for a purpose help to ensure the type and consistency of information collected and recorded about a patient's care. They also help to ensure the completeness and accuracy of patient records.

### Patient records

Patient records are a vital method of communication among professionals in all practice settings. Verbal dialogue between the professions often arises from the documented patient record. Patient records may be handwritten or generated using information technology. This section will consider handwritten patient records, with a later section considering electronic records. The general principles for handwritten and electronic records and record keeping are the same. Box 5.4 provides some guidelines on how good record keeping can be developed.

## BOX 5.4
### Record keeping – good-practice guidelines

- Always ensure records are factual, consistent and accurate and written chronologically

- Ensure your hand writing is legible

- Avoid using jargon, abbreviations, meaningless phrases, irrelevant speculation, offensive comments and colloquialisms

- Only record relevant information

- All entries must be signed with your name and job title printed alongside the first entry

- Make sure that you accurately date and time all records as close to the actual time as possible

- Always record information as soon as possible after the event has occurred

- Records must be written in language that the patient or client will be able to understand

- Never alter or destroy any records without being authorized to do so

- Any alterations must be crossed out with one line, dated, timed and signed.

- Black ink should be used to ensure that the records are readable if photocopied or scanned.

**Note:** Remember that any information you record may be scrutinized at a later date.

Adapted from Record Keeping Guidance for Nurses and Midwives (NMC, 2010)

Adherence to the Record Keeping Standard is crucial to ensure that patients / clients receive high quality care. The death of Leo Norris by his mother, who was suffering from severe post-natal depression, tragically highlights the consequences of poor record keeping by those professionals involved in the care of the mother and baby Leo. Box 5.5 shows some of the Recommendations related to information sharing that were made to the agencies and health and social care professionals involved in this case.

## BOX 5.5

**The report into the death of Leo Norris (Torbay Safeguarding Children Board, *Serious Case Review*, 2010)**
This had a significant number of recommendations, for various agencies, that focused on written and verbal communication including the following:

**Recommendation 8.4 – Inter-agency recommendations**
To support practitioners in providing safe care for children Torbay Safeguarding Children Board (SCB) should ensure that all safeguarding training, both single agency and inter-agency, clarifies the

circumstances when the need for information sharing to safeguard children and unborn babies takes precedence over the duty of confidentiality to adults. It should emphasize the importance of comprehensive documentation of decisions, the reasons for decisions and actions taken.

### Recommendation 9.3 – Torbay Care Trust - Health Visiting
### Record Keeping

Practitioners need to be aware of the Record Keeping Standard and adhere to it at all times.

Records must be contemporaneous, legible, dated, timed and signed by the practitioner which is identifiable by their signed and printed names

All records should contain the reason for contact, a plan of care, outcomes and reviewing arrangements

Records should reflect all conversations with other professionals, including the 'corridor conversations' identified within this review.

Ongoing Record Keeping Audits are essential to ensure compliance with the standard, and to inform any training that is required.

### Communication

A process must be implemented whereby all Specialist Community Public Health Practitioners meet regularly with GPs and Midwives to discuss families of concern. Where appropriate this forum should be opened to partner agencies such as mental health services.

Patients' notes provide an important channel of communication as they ensure that a patient's treatment and care can be maintained if the relevant professional (for example, doctor, nurse, occupational therapist, health visitor, school nurse, pharmacist, social worker) cannot be found or if there is insufficient time to contact them. Although patient records are absolutely vital for the provision of high-quality care, they should not be seen as a substitute for two-way face-to-face synchronous communication.

## Reflective activity

This exercise will introduce you to the audit of record keeping. Select three sets of records in which you have recently documented entries. Using the record keeping guidance from your professional body complete an audit of your own records. You might find it useful to work through your record keeping with your mentor or colleague. Consider the following questions:

- Are all your entries legible?
- Are all your entries dated and timed?
- Did you print your name and job title alongside your initial entry?
- Are your entries made in chronological order?
- Was the patient / client involved in making the entries to their record?
- Have you used any unexplained acronyms, abbreviations or terminology?
- Have you included any irrelevant information?
- Would other health and social care professionals understand what you have written?
- If you have made changes to your entries have you made them clearly?

Patient records are covered by a number of Acts of Parliament, including the Data Protection Act 1998, the Human Rights Act 1998 and the Freedom of Information Act 2000. All health and social care professionals should familiarize themselves with the salient points of each Act.

## EVIDENCE BASE

- Go to the website **http://www.dh.gov.uk/** Read the document Records Management: NHS Code of Practice.
- Go to the website **http://www.ico.gov.uk/** Read the Data Protection Act 1998.
- Go to the website **http://www.ico.gov.uk/for_organizations/freedom_of_information. aspx** Read the Freedom of information Act 2000

## TYPES OF MEETINGS

Effective team communication is essential if interprofessional working is to be successful. Types of meetings that promote team communication include:

1 team/staff meetings
2 multidisciplinary team meetings
3 child protection case conferences.

## TEAM MEETINGS

Team meetings, sometimes referred to as staff meetings, is a term used to refer to semi-formal meetings which are held in most practice environments on a regular basis. These meetings are usually chaired by the team leader/ head of department/service manager.

Team meetings provide the opportunity for the team leader and team members to meet and discuss matters that affect the team. These meetings provide a two-way communication channel between the team leader and the team members and serve multiple purposes. They provide an opportunity for the team leader to share information with the team, such as issues related to the organization in which they are working. Sharing information that affects the whole organization and not just information related to the team makes the team members feel they are valued by the organization and enhances their loyalty to the overall organization and to the team.

Team meetings also enable team members to make suggestions and comments to the team leader about the ways in which the team could enhance its practice. This two-way channel of communication also enables the team leader to share with the team information that will affect the day-to-day activities of the team. If, for example, the team leader wishes to implement a change to the working practices of the team, the team meeting provides an appropriate place for this discussion to take place. All team members will be present and they can all participate in the debate and decision-making process. Commitment to any proposed changes can be increased if the team leader involves the team members in this process. Even if some of the team members do not agree with the final decision that has been made, they have had the opportunity to air their views and can understand the context within which the decision has been made.

Team meetings also bring the whole team together and although they are not primarily a social occasion, there will be opportunities for the team members to chat informally, for example before the meeting starts, during the coffee/tea break and after the meeting has finished.

The opportunity for team members to meet on a regular basis to communicate face to face with each other and the team leader is essential if the team is to function effectively. Team meetings are, however, particularly important for those teams where the professionals spend a large proportion of their time working alone, for example, members of the palliative-care team or primary health care team.

Successful team meetings do not just happen and in the next section we will discuss the various steps that should be taken to increase the chances of holding an effective team meeting.

## Skills required for a successful team meeting

There are a number of elements that need to be considered in order to ensure that the team meeting achieves something. These elements apply to all meetings and not just team meetings. There are three elements:

1 preparation
2 the meeting
3 after the meeting

### Preparation

Preparation is the key to a successful meeting and it is the team leader who will take on this responsibility. There are a number of decisions that the team leader will have to make, including:

- **When to hold the meeting** – If the meeting is to be a regular meeting, rather than a one off, it is best if the meeting is held on the same day, at the same time and at the same frequency, for example, the first Thursday of each month between 9.30 a.m. and 11.00 a.m. The frequency of this will depend on the type of meeting; for some meetings once a month may be appropriate, for others bi-monthly and for other meetings once a fortnight may be considered necessary.

  Commitment to attending a team meeting is higher if the meeting has a regular 'slot' in the calendar. This is because staff know in advance when the meeting is going to take place and can schedule other work commitments around the meeting.

- **Where to hold the meeting** – Choosing the right location for the meeting is essential. The venue should be easy for all members to reach, with adequate car-parking facilities. The room should be the right size for the number of staff expected to attend and tea/coffee-making facilities should be readily accessible. Get it wrong – venue difficult to find; no tea/coffee available; no car parking; room too small – then staff will be very reluctant to attend another meeting.

  With agreement of all the team members, it may be considered appropriate to rotate the venue of the meeting. In a primary health care team, for example, where the team may be geographically widely dispersed, rotating the venue will mean that it is not always the same members of the team travelling the longest distances. Rotating the venue, where appropriate, will increase the attendance at meetings, as no member of the team will feel that they are always being disadvantaged by having to travel a long distance.

- **Setting the agenda** – The agenda gives the meeting a structure and focus. From the agenda the team members will know why they are meeting and what they will be discussing. The purpose of the meeting, for example, might be to share information; problem solve; make decisions; or for planning and coordinating the work of the team.

It is the team leader's responsibility to set the agenda. The agenda should be set to ensure that it keeps all team members interested and involved, while making sure that the purpose of the meeting is achieved. It is important that items for an agenda are not just generated by the team leader but that team members also contribute items. If team members have contributed to the setting of the agenda, they should feel that they have an important role in the meeting and that the team leader values their contributions to the effective functioning of the team. Box 5.6 illustrates a typical agenda.

## BOX 5.6

**East Street palliative-care team meeting**
To be held at Hawthorne House, Wednesday, 22 March 2013, 9.30 a.m. to 11.00 a.m.

**AGENDA**

1 Apologies for absence

2 Minutes of the previous meeting (08.03.2013)

3 Matters arising

4 Proposed changes to the referral process (Paper 1 – attached)

5 Student placements within the palliative care team (Paper 2 – attached)

6 Office space at Napier House

7 Organization of social event for the team

8 Any other business

9 Date of next meeting.

The team leader needs to give consideration to the order that items appear on the agenda. Typically, essential business items should be at the beginning of the agenda. In the specimen agenda, the crucial business item is the discussion related to the proposed changes to the referral process. The agenda should close with items that are not controversial and celebrate the success of the team. In the specimen agenda, the last topic identified for discussion is the organization of a social event for the team. This item should ensure that the meeting closes on a high note.

The agenda and any relevant papers must be circulated to all the team members in advance of the meeting. This will enable the team members to prepare for the meeting. Team members have the responsibility to:

- On receiving the agenda and accompanying papers, check and note the day, date, time and venue for the meeting in their diary.
- Let the team leader know as soon as possible if they are able to attend or not. It is important that if a team member is not able to attend they send their apologies to the team leader.
- Ensure that prior to the meeting they have read the minutes from the previous meeting. Team members must be prepared to provide an update on any action point that they have been asked to address.
- Ensure that prior to the meeting they have read any relevant papers or documents so that they can contribute knowledgeably to the discussion.

## The meeting

The success of a meeting will depend on how the meeting is chaired and the quality of the contributions that individual team members make during the discussions. To help facilitate successful meetings it is useful if the team agree some team ground rules. For example:

- be prepared for the meeting
- come to the meeting on time
- start and end the meeting on time
- respect and value the diversity of team members
- participate in the meeting
- actively listen to the discussions
- make decisions by consensus.

**Role of the chairperson during the meeting** This is a demanding role and the success or otherwise of the meeting will depend to a large extent on whether the chair carries out their role effectively. During the meeting the chair has a number of responsibilities:

- **Opening the meeting** – It is important to start the meeting on time and with introductions if necessary. If everybody in the room does not know each other, it is important that everyone introduces themselves. It is also good practice to remind the members of the group of the purpose of the meeting and, if appropriate, housekeeping arrangements (for example, location of fire exits; toilets; tea- and coffee-making facilities) and the team ground rules. The chairperson may also ask if the team are happy with the order of the items on the agenda and changes to the order can be made at this point in the meeting if considered appropriate

- **Encouraging participation** – It is important that all group members participate in the debate. The chair will need to encourage everyone to join in; some members will need more direct encouragement than others. Using open questions, for example, 'What do you think about the proposed changes in the referral process?' is more likely to facilitate discussion than a closed question, for example, 'How much money has been spent on photocopying this month?' Closed questions are, however, useful if the chair requires specific information from the group

- **Encouraging decision making** – Making decisions is an essential part of the meeting. The chair will encourage the team to make decisions. In facilitating a decision, the chair will actively listen to the debate, drawing together the threads of the debate and summarizing the points made by the team. If appropriate, the chair will help to clarify points and ask pertinent questions of the team if there appear to be key areas of the debate that have not been explored. It is also important that the chair does not allow the team to wander off the point and that he or she ensures that if disagreements occur these are fully explored by the team before a decision is made. Decisions should be made by consensus of all the team members.

**Role of the team members** A team member has the responsibility to participate in the debate and air their views on the topic being discussed. When contributing to the discussions, it is important that ideas are clearly and precisely presented. This will ensure that thoughts are effectively communicated. It is important that the team member does not become emotive about the issues that they are discussing as this will detract from the overall point that is being made. Meetings will be successful if all team members contribute, respect and value the contributions that other team members are making to the discussion, and actively listen to each other's contributions.

**Role of the minute taker** It is important that minutes are taken at meetings as they form an agreed record of the discussions and decisions made at the meeting. The minutes not only record the decisions that have been made but also the action points that arise from the decision, that is, how, by whom and by when the decision is going to be implemented. At future meetings, minutes can be used to review the progress of the work of the team.

## After the meeting

Even after the meeting has finished, there are a number of tasks that the chair, team members and minute taker must complete to ensure the meeting was a success.

**Role of the chairperson**  Following the meeting the chairperson should evaluate the meeting with the intention of improving future meetings. The following series of questions could be used as a framework for undertaking this evaluation:

- Did the meeting start and end on time?
- Was the purpose of the meeting clear?
- Did all team members contribute to the meeting?
- Did the team work toward consensus?
- Did the team identify by whom, by when and how decisions were going to be implemented?
- Was sufficient time available to debate all the issues fully?
- Was all the necessary paperwork available for the meeting?

**Role of the team members**  After the meeting, the team members must ensure that any action point they are responsible for is implemented within the timescale identified at the meeting.

**Role of the minute taker**  The minutes from a meeting should be written up as soon as possible after the meeting has finished. The final draft of the minutes should be checked for accuracy with the chair. Minutes should be circulated to all the members of the team who attended the meeting, and to those members who sent their apologies. This type of circulation list ensures that all team members are kept informed of what was achieved at the meeting.

# MULTIDISCIPLINARY TEAM (MDT) MEETING

There are many similarities between multidisciplinary team (MDT) meetings and team meetings. This section will therefore focus on the unique challenges of developing effective MDT meetings.

MDT membership is developed around the patient's journey through the system to ensure that all relevant professionals are able to play an active role in the care of the patient.

The following tables are three examples of MDTs and their typical membership. Table 5.1 shows a Stroke MDT and Table 5.2 shows a Breast cancer MDT.

| Table 5.1   Stroke MDT | |
| --- | --- |
| • Medical staff | • Social worker |
| • Nursing staff | • Dietician |
| • Specialist stroke nurse | • Stroke coordinator |
| • Occupational therapist | • Clinical psychologist |
| • Physiotherapists | • Family and carer support coordinator |
| • Speech and language therapists | • MDT coordinator |

| Table 5.2   Breast cancer  MDT | |
| --- | --- |
| • Radiologist | • MDT coordinator |
| • Oncologist | • Nursing staff |
| • Histopathologist | • Diagnostic radiographer |
| • Specialist colo-rectal | • Surgeon |
| • Therapeutic radiographer | • Plastic surgeon |
| • Clinical nurse specialist | |

Table 5.3 shows a Children's Network MDT that has been set up in the Borough of Haringey, London. The purpose of the MDT is to deliver support for children, young people and families through a more integrated and joined-up approach, with staff working in partnership with staff in a range of settings to deliver the 'team around the child'. This is an excellent example of interprofessional working across three sectors: social services, education and health.

| Table 5.3   Children's network  MDT | |
| --- | --- |
| • Education psychologists | • Early years practitioners |
| • Education welfare officers | • Teenage pregnancy and parenthood officers |
| • Behavioural support teachers | • Parent support advisors |
| • Language support teachers | • Family support workers |
| • Autism teachers | • Other staff delivering targeted support to children and young people, e.g. health professionals |

As these three examples illustrate, the number of different professionals involved in one MDT can be in excess of ten people and this provides unique challenges for developing effective MDT meetings.

# What are the challenges for MDT meetings?

The challenges for developing effective communication channels for an MDT meeting can be divided into three broad areas:

1 coordinating the MDT meeting
2 time commitment
3 resources

## Coordinating the MDT meeting

MDTs will normally have an MDT coordinator who will provide administrative/secretarial support before, during and after the MDT meeting. The MDT co-ordinator is crucial to the smooth running of the MDT meeting and to streamlining the patient pathway. The key responsibilities of the coordinator include:

- arranging the meeting
- obtaining the list of patients to be discussed at the meeting
- getting the patient's details, for example, patients notes, imaging, histopathology reports
- recording attendance at the meetings
- recording decisions made about a patient's/client's treatment and management on the MDT *pro forma*
- booking and tracking appointments and tests for patients
- ensuring effective communication between the MDT and its related teams in primary, secondary and tertiary care.

The MDT coordinator is therefore at the hub of the MDT and is of crucial importance to effective communications between core members of the MDT, members of the extended MDT and the patient. The MDT coordinator must possess excellent verbal and written communication skills, which can be adapted and applied to the broad-ranging situations they will meet.

## Time commitment

The majority of MDTs meet on a weekly basis and meetings are usually scheduled for 60–90 minutes. Core members or their agreed cover are expected to attend the majority of meetings. Although the actual MDT meeting may only last for 90 minutes, members need time to make sure that all the relevant images have been reviewed in advance of the meeting. Time is also required after the meeting to carry out any tasks resulting from decisions taken at the MDT meeting. As people may be members of many MDTs, the time commitment for individuals will not be insignificant.

## Resources

To facilitate the effective functioning of an MDT meeting, specific resources are made available. The meeting room will have image-viewing equipment and equipment for viewing pathology slides. This means that all members of the

MDT can view the patient information at the same time, allowing each member to make their own unique contribution to the discussion about the patient's treatment and management plan.

Another resource that can aid the communication process at an MDT meeting is the availability of a laptop computer with projection facilities. This facility enables the MDT coordinator to type decisions made directly onto the MDT pro forma, which can then be viewed and agreed by those members present. At end of the MDT meeting, therefore, all the decisions made have been electronically recorded and agreed as accurate. The decisions from the MDT meeting can then be communicated electronically to all relevant parties, for example, members of the MDT, the patient's GP, palliative-care team, within 24 hours.

Video conferencing facilities are another resource that can aid communication between members of the MDT. This resource is invaluable as it allows for cross-site communication, allowing core members from different sites to participate in the MDT meeting without needing to spend time on travelling.

As can be seen, an MDT meeting may use the entire range of communication methods: face to face, telephone, written, e-mail, video conferencing and IT equipment, to enhance the effective working of the MDT. This should result in the patient receiving the most suitable care from diagnosis through treatment to follow-up care and support with the least delay. This will contribute to improved patient outcome.

## Health care professional

Hannah, a senior occupational therapist, discusses her perceptions of the multi-disciplinary meetings that she attends:

My experience and perception of attending MDT meetings and how they work has changed dramatically as my career has progressed.

As an inexperienced 'novice' band 5, just starting out in my OT career, my perception of MDT meetings was that they took place to discuss a patient caseload and their progress in recovery. They were led and chaired by consultants (doctors), in line with the medical model. Each professional contributed their opinion when requested and if your opinion didn't match that of the consultant then your views could be dismissed. As an inexperienced practitioner I had little confidence to speak up and contest the decisions made that weren't in line with my findings.

As an experienced 'expert' band 7, 12 years on, my perception of MDT meetings is now very different. More recently I have experienced MDT meetings with the purpose of reviewing service development initiatives. These are often chaired and led by an allied health professional, such as myself, even when consultants and matrons are in attendance. With confidence in my opinions and views, I now feel able to speak out and debate against the opinions of others in order to gain the best outcomes for patients, regardless of hierarchy.

In today's NHS the value of MDT meetings in any sense cannot be underestimated and each profession should feel confident to express their opinion in order to progress the patient though the health care system and ensure services are designed to meet their needs, despite 'power relations'.

# CHILD PROTECTION CASE CONFERENCES

A child protection case conference is a critical part of the process of safe-guarding children and will take place if there is a concern that a child is believed to have been harmed, or to be at significant risk of being harmed. This harm will involve one or more of the following categories: physical abuse; sexual abuse; emotional abuse and neglect. The purpose of the conference is:

1 to share information regarding the child's development needs, the parents' or carers' capacity to meet these needs and to ensure the child's safety

2 to consider the evidence presented to the conference in context of all the information provided and make a judgement about the likelihood of the child suffering significant harm in the future and whether the child is continuing to, or is likely to, suffer significant harm

3 to decide what future action is required to safeguard and promote the welfare of the child.

*Shabde and Buckland (2010, p. 571)*

A conference is attended by those professionals involved with the current care of the child as well as the child's parent / carers. The following table gives the typical membership of a conference.

| Table 5.4   Child protection case conference | |
|---|---|
| • Local authority children's social worker | • Health visitor |
| • Family / child's GP | • Professionals involved with the parents, e.g family support services; adult services |
| • Family members (including wider family) | • Foster carers |
| • Child dependinng on their age | • Staff in youth justice system |
| • School public health nurse | • Police |
| • Teaching staff | • Residential care staff |
| • Paediatricians | • Midwife |

As Table 5.4 illustrates, a conference has a large number of different professionals and agencies involved and this provides unique challenges for effective interprofessional collaboration.

### Health care professional

Jenny, a senior health visitor talks about her experiences of attending child protection conferences.

" *A child protection conference is probably the most important interprofessional meeting that a health visitor will be involved in. The conference is called whenever a child is a subject of a significant level of concern. The level of concern will usually be high, however, the quality of the evidence does not have to stand the rigorous scrutiny of a court. It is sufficient that one or more persons involved with the child wants to share that concern with the professional team, the meeting will decide what action, if any, to take.*

" *Membership consists of all agencies that can be involved with the child and their family and carers. Health is represented by a health visitor and a general practitioner and if the child is of school age a school nurse and a member of the teaching team. The police will be represented at initial conferences but only at review meetings if they have a specific role. The conference will be chaired by either a senior social worker or an independent chair, depending on the area. The chair has a coordination and communication role.*

" *Open communication is a core principle, which can challenge some assumptions that professionals work with. The police are often concerned not to disrupt or harm an investigation by risking that an offender becomes aware of their interest or has the chance to dispose of evidence. They must accept that protection of a vulnerable person takes precedence over the conviction of an offender. Health professionals have to accept that confidentiality can and must be breached if protection is an aim. This is the case even if it threatens the relationship with a service user. Education professionals are often reluctant to be seen as supporting social agencies that enforce criminal or civil law, such as the police and social services, but as with all others they must accept that priority responsibilities exist. Social workers are guided by valid and espoused values and these again have to be ordered in priority such that the right of a child to be safe is more important than an adult having to face anxiety when their behaviour is reasonably questioned.*

" *The meeting is democratic in that each member's voice has to be heard and each different professional perspective respected. A 'public level of evidence' is normally accepted. This means reasonable suspicion is sufficient to act. Members try and avoid common value judgements that are applied in society and discrimination on the usual inappropriate grounds with particular concern for alternative lifestyle issues. Judgement has to be made on the principle of exposure to, or potential exposure to, harm for those who cannot protect themselves.*

" *My experience is that case conferences require openness, a willingness to listen to other professionals and a personal insight into the social values each member learns as a consequence of their professional role. The emotional experiences shared can be quite threatening to the less experienced and perhaps naive professional who forgets the person within the professional role. The need for the person to share thoughts and feelings candidly and openly in a trusting and empathetic forum is essential. Intuitive reasoning comes from sub-acute awareness and conferences are attended by persons who all have a part of the puzzle*

*(Continued)*

*but not all. Sharing those parts and the thoughts and feelings that are raised as a consequence of partial understanding is a core part of the process. If one person has a different perspective to the others that does not mean they are wrong. Every individual view has to be assimilated into each member's understanding. No person has to agree with all views, only appreciate how and why they are held and that requires interprofessional empathy. This has to be learned maturely through personal insights.*

## EVIDENCE BASE

To find out more about child protection case conferences read the following article:

● Shabde, N. and Buckland, A. (2010) Attending a child protection conference – a paediatrician's contribution. *Paediatrics and Child Health*, **20** (12): 571–576.

● Go to the websites:

  ● http://www.clacksweb.org.uk/site/documents/childcare/childprotec tioncaseconferenceinformationleaflets/ and read the child protection case conference leaflets for parents/carer and for children and young people.

  ● http://www.playfieldinstitute.co.uk/ and read the information provided for practitioners attending child protection case conferences.

## ENABLING TECHNOLOGIES

Traditionally, the transfer of information between health care professionals, patients and other agencies has relied upon letters or telephone calls and much of the transfer has relied on information carried by patients. In the 21st century, the new information technologies are being used and developed to enable information to be shared effectively between teams and organizations.

In April 2005, NHS Connecting for Health, part of the Department of Health Informatics Directorate, was launched. Its primary role was to deliver the National Programme for IT, which was set up to provide a range of centralized services and applications to help modernize the NHS and improve the quality of patient care. In 2011, following the change of government and consequent NHS reforms, it was announced that the National Programme for IT would no longer be run as a national, centralized programme and that decision making and responsibility for NHS information technology would be taken at a local level.

However, the established services and applications, which have already provided benefits to patients will be built upon and continue to be delivered, these include:

● Spine
● N3 Network
● NHSmail

- Secondary Uses Services
- Summary Care Records (electronic health records)
- Choose and Book Service
- Electronic Prescription Service
- Picture Archiving and Communications Systems (PACS)

In this section, we will discuss two of these services and applications, electronic records and PACS, and consider how these technologies will enhance interprofessional working.

## Electronic health records

Patient records are the key to the delivery of high-quality health and social care. There are numerous government documents and reports that highlight the necessity for single interprofessional patient records that can be accessed by the patient and all those professionals caring for them. These documents include *Essence of Care* (Department of Health, 2003b), the *National Service Framework for Older People* (Department of Health, 2001), the *Victoria Climbié Enquiry* (Secretary of State for Health, 2003), *Our Health, our care, our say: a new direction for community services* (Department of Health, 2006) and *Patient Safety* (House of Commons Health Committee, 2009). Electronic records will facilitate the implementation of interprofessional single-patient records. There are three types of electronic health records:

1 Summary Care Record (SCR)

   This is designed to provide a summary of clinical information that would be useful in the event of urgent or unscheduled care for a patient. It is created from the records of organizations already delivering care to a patient. The information is initially derived from the patient's GP record and will contain details of medication, adverse reactions and allergies. The record will be held nationally and can be looked at anywhere in the NHS in England and is designed to improve the safety, quality and efficiency of patient care.

   SCRs were first introduced in 2009 and by 2011 over ten million (1.25 per cent) patients had a SCR, with a pledge that the 34 million people that had been written to about the SCR would have a record created by March 2013 at the latest (Gutteridge, 2011).

   Patients can electronically access their Summary Care Record via a secure web service called HealthSpace which provides two levels of service to patients:

   a) Basic self-registration service which provides patients with an online personal organizer; a calendar to record information and a facility to find doctors, dentists and other NHS services.

   b) Advanced service, which provides patients with access to their Summary Care Record and HealthSpace Communicator, which is a secure way for patients to communicate electronically with health care staff.

**2** Detailed care record

This is a longitudinal record held in primary care that contains a note of any contact with health services during the life of the patient.

**3** Records held in prescriptions, referrals and other local systems

It is important that health and social care professionals are aware of the legal aspects of working with electronic records. All the Acts of Parliament that apply to manual records also apply to electronic records. These are the Data Protection Act 1998; the Access to Health Records Act 1990 and the Freedom of Information Act 2000. There are, however, additional considerations that need to be given to the management of electronic records, which include the use, storage, security and retrieval of records and compliance with the Computer Misuse Act 1990, the Electronic Communications Act 2000 and the Communications Act 2003. All health and social care professionals should familiarize themselves with these additional requirements for the handling of electronic records.

## EVIDENCE BASE

Go to website http://www.dh.gov.uk/ and read the document 'Records Management: NHS Code of Practice'.

Go to website http://www.connectingforhealth.nhs.uk/systemsandservices/infogov/codes/securitycode.pdf and read the document 'Information Security Management: NHS Code of Practice'.

There can be no doubt that the introduction of electronic health records will enhance communication across an interprofessional team. Electronic records are easier to read, less bulky and reduce the need for professionals to re-record information that has already been recorded by another professional. A good example of information that is duplicated if profession-specific records are maintained is the patient's medical history. How often do we ask a patient a question about their medical history to be asked, 'Don't you all talk to each other? I told the nurse/doctor/physiotherapist that'.

Over the next few years the NHS care records service will be linking up electronic records, both within one particular organization and also with other organizations where a patient may receive care, such as hospitals, clinics and GP practices. This will mean that all members of the interprofessional team caring for that patient will have access to the information about the patient's care, where and when the professional needs it, using a secure computer system.

Electronic health records will, therefore be invaluable to all interprofessional teams, but particularly for those teams that are geographically dispersed, for example primary-care teams.

## Electronic social care records (ESCR)

The ESCR was introduced in 2003 to provide social care users with a good consistent service from all government organizations. The ESCR, like the electronic health record, aims to bring together all the relevant information for the service user into one place. Three types of information are held on the ESCR:

1 Structured information, for example:

- national forms, such as those used for recording children's information
- local forms
- forms completed by service users, such as self-referral or financial assessment forms.

2 Unstructured information which covers all other recordings, for example:

- letters
- emails
- records of telephone calls
- meetings notes
- video clips.

3 Coded data, which is mainly for management and statistical reports

*Department of Health (2003c)*

The introduction of electronic health records and electronic social care records has resulted in a single assessment process being introduced, not just for the older person (Department of Health, 2001), but for all service users. This integration of health and social care systems will enhance inteprofess-sional working between health and social care practitioners and will lead to an enhanced quality of service being provided to the service user.

## EVIDENCE BASE

Go to website **http://www.dh.gov** and read the document 'National Electronic Social Care Record Survey Report 2006/07'.

## Picture archiving and communication systems (PACS)

PACS is a system which captures, stores, distributes and displays static or moving digital images such as radiographs, CT, ultrasound, MR, nuclear medicine. The system takes away any need to print on film and to file or distribute images manually. PACS is well embedded in day-to-day clinical practice across all acute trusts in England.

The benefits of PACS for effective interprofessional working and the consequent enhancement of patient care are several. As PACS stores images digitally, it means that the images can be distributed to any number of workstations simultaneously. This allows team members to view the same information across one or more locations at the same time, enabling more discussion and collaborative working to the benefit of the patient.

PACS are ideal for use during multidisciplinary team meetings (MDTs). As each patient is discussed, the relevant images can be retrieved and displayed so that the entire MDT can view them at the same time. As a result, the use of PACs means that the discussion and decisions about a patient's treatment and care plan are fully informed by information provided by the images. As PACS is a central database, it also means that if a patient has had images taken at a different NHS Trust to where they are currently being treated, the images can also be retrieved instantaneously. There is no longer the need to wait for images to arrive from another hospital or to rely on patients carrying packets of film around the hospital and between sites during the course of their care.

PACS also enables clinicians to access specialist opinion from anywhere within the NHS across England, that is, the acute, primary-care and community settings. The benefits to the patient are evident, no longer does the patient have to be living in a particular part of England to have specialist input into their treatment and care plan. For the professionals involved in the discussions with the specialist, it provides an interprofessional learning opportunity.

It is clear to see that PACS has enhanced interprofessional learning and interprofessional working between health care professionals. For the patient, their experience of the care they receive is considerably enhanced, culminating in improved care planning and possibly quicker discharge from hospital.

## WHAT ARE THE BARRIERS TO INTERPROFESSIONAL COMMUNICATION?

In the previous sections we have considered verbal and written methods of communication and enabling technologies as ways in which interprofessional communication and therefore interprofessional working can be enhanced. However, the effectiveness of these communication methods and technologies depends entirely on the communication skills of the individual professional and the context within which they are working. The communication process is illustrated in Figure 5.1.

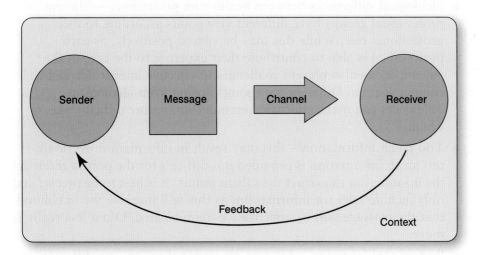

Figure 5.1   The communication process
Adapted from http://www.mindtools.com and used with permission.

Barriers to communication can occur at any stage of the communication process and have the potential to create misunderstandings and confusion. As a health and social care professional, it is important that you have an awareness of the possible barriers to communication and at what point these may occur in the communication process. This will enable you to take the appropriate steps to break down the barriers and deliver your information effectively.

There are many potential barriers to communication including:

- **Inappropriate channel of communication selected** – for example, selecting a written method when face-to-face communication would have been better or vice versa.

- **Distractions** – for example, other people talking, equipment, noise, televisions, radios, interruptions.

- **Hierarchy** – the hierarchal nature of health care creates power gaps that contribute to less than optimal communication between different professionals and with patients (see Chapter 7).

- **Lack of time** – to communicate effectively takes time, and the pressures of the workplace may result in the health care professionals doing another task or thinking about what they are going to do next at the same time as a message is being communicated to them. As a consequence, the health care professional is not fully concentrating and focusing on the person speaking and this may result in vital information being lost or misinterpreted.

- **Complex messages** – communication within and between professionals is often complex and as a result frequently lengthy. A complex lengthy message will increase the chances of the message being misunderstood or misinterpreted.

- **Ideological differences between health care professions** – different professional groups have different viewpoints according to their professional role. While this may be viewed positively, as each professional is able to contribute their expertise to the care of the patient, it can also present challenges to effective interprofessional communication. Different viewpoints arising from ideological differences can make effective communication more difficult (see Chapter 7).

- **Too much information** – this may result in information overload. If too much information is provided it is difficult for the person receiving the information to extract the salient points. It is best to be precise and only include relevant information, as this will increase the likelihood that the message will be effectively communicated. Often less really is more.

- **Professional language** – different professional groups use different professional language, which can lead to problems of understanding each other (see Chapter 7).

**Jargon**
Technical or specialized language associated with a particular profession

- **Professional jargon** – professionals frequently use jargon when communicating with patients. This is likely to result in the patient receiving incomplete information because they are unable to understand all the information being communicated by the professional.

- **Too many communications** – in busy and complex environments, such as those found in health care, a health care professional will receive numerous communications on a daily basis. These communications may be via the telephone or e-mail or during a ward round or team meeting. With so many communications, it can be difficult, if not impossible, to determine which communications are most critical.

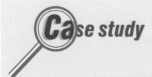 **Case study**

### Exploring barriers to effective communication

You are at the nurses' station on the ward completing paperwork. A relative of one of your patients comes to the nurses' station and is clearly anxious about their relative. They wish to discuss the care of their relative with you. The telephone rings and you are the only member of staff around.

With reference to the case study:

- What are the barriers to communication that exist in this scenario?

- How could you overcome these barriers?

- How would you deal with this situation?

## KEY POINTS

The potential barriers to communication are:

- distractions
- hierarchy
- inappropriate channel of communication
- too many communications
- complex messages
- professional language
- too much information
- ideological differences between different professionals
- lack of time.

## RAPID RECAP

Check your progress so far by working through each of the following questions.

1 What are the main methods of verbal communication?

2 What are the benefits of multidisciplinary team meetings?

3 How do electronic health records and electronic social care records enhance interprofessional communication?

4 What factors inhibit interprofessional communication?

If you have difficulty with more than one of the questions, read through the section again to refresh your understanding before moving on.

## REFERENCES

Chapman, A. (2012) Mehrabian's communication research. [online] Available at http://www.business balls.com/mehrabiancommunications.htm. Accessed August 2012.

Department of Health (2000) The NHS Plan: A plan for investment, a plan for reform. London: HMSO.

Department of Health (2001) National service framework for older people. London: HMSO.

Department of Health (2003a) Guiding principles relating to the commissioning and provision of communication. Leeds: Department of Health.

Department of Health (2003b) Essence of care: patient-focused benchmarking for health care practitioners. London: HMSO.

Department of Health (2003c) Defining the electronic social care record. London: Information Policy Unit – Social Care.

Department of Health (2006) *Our health, our care, our say: a new direction for community services.* London: COI.

Gutteridge, C. (2011) *Clinical use of the summary care record.* Available from: **www.connectingfor health.nhs.uk**

Haringey Local Safeguarding Board (2009) *Serious case review: Baby Peter.* Available from **http://www.har ingeylscb.org/executive_summary_peter_final.pdf.**

Healthcare Inspectorate Wales (2009) *Report of a review in respect of Mr D and the provision of mental health services, following the homicide of Father Paul committed in March 2007.* Available from **www.hiw.org.uk**

House of Commons Health Committee (2009) *Patient safety.* London: The Stationery Office.

Nursing and Midwifery Council (2010) *Record keeping guidance for nurses and midwives.* London: NMC.

Secretary of State for Health (2001) *Learning from Bristol.* London: The Stationery Office.

Secretary of State for Health (2003) *The Victoria Climbié Inquiry.* London: The Stationery Office.

Shabde, N. and Buckland, A. (2010) Attending a child protection conference – a paediatrician's contribution. *Paediatrics and Child Health.* **20** (12) 571–576.

Torbay Safeguarding Children Board (2010) *Serious Case Review.* Available from **www.torbay.gov.uk/ c18-execsumm.pdf.**

# CHAPTER 6

# INTERPROFESSIONAL LEARNING WITHIN A PRACTICE ENVIRONMENT

## LEARNING OBJECTIVES

*By the end of this chapter you should be able to:*

● Discuss the developments in interprofessional learning

● Understand situated learning theory

● Create a learning environment within which effective interprofessional learning can take place

● Critically appraise the concept of interprofessional mentorship.

## INTRODUCTION

The tragic deaths of young children, such as the children undergoing heart surgery at Bristol Royal Infirmary (Secretary of State for Health, 2001), Victoria Climbié (Secretary of State for Health, 2003) and Baby Peter (Laming, 2009) and the untimely deaths of Father Paul Bennett (Health care Inspectorate Wales, 2009) and Leo Norris (Torbay Safeguarding Children Board, Serious Case Review, 2010) due to lapses in mental health care, indicate that despite all of the rhetoric, health and social care professionals, whether working in the statutory, voluntary or private sectors are still not effectively collaborating. The reports into these deaths have suggested both implicitly and explicitly that 'shared learning' is one of the key methods by which collaboration could be cultivated and encouraged.

There can be no doubt, as the reports into these tragic deaths so vividly illustrate, that effective interprofessional collaboration between health and social care professionals will enhance the patient outcome. But is 'interprofessional education' the panacea that we have been searching for to facilitate effective interprofessional working? The fundamental questions that still need to be addressed are:

- Does interprofessional education actually enhance interprofessional working?
- Does interprofessional education actually enhance patient outcomes?

As yet, we do not know the answer to these questions but progress is being made in evidencing improvements in professional practice and patient care as a result of exposure to interprofessional education (Reeves *et al.*, 2010). A number of systematic reviews of interprofessional education research have been conducted during the last decade (Zwarenstein *et al.*, 1999; Cooper *et al.*, 2001; Barr *et al.*, 2005; Freeth *et al.*, 2005; Hammick *et al.*, 2007; Reeves *et al.*, 2010) and these have indicated the positive impact of inter-professional education. These include changes in learner's attitudes towards one another's professions, improvements in knowledge of interprofessional collaboration, enhancement of collaborative behaviour and improvements in the delivery of patient care.

However, the latest Cochrane systematic undertaken by Reeves *et al.* (2010), like the earlier one carried out by Zwarenstein *et al.* (1999), still found that the interprofessional education research studies lacked the meth-odological rigour needed to convincingly understand the impact of interpro-fessional education on professional practice and/or health care outcomes.

We will begin this chapter by discussing the UK health and social care policies and professional developments that have influenced the develop-ments of **interprofessional learning**. Next, we will examine the learning theories that have been applied to interprofessional education and the creation of a learning environment within which effective interprofessional learning can be engendered. Finally, we will consider the importance of supporting learners within the practice environment. Mentorship and in particular interprofes-sional mentorship and how this role might be further developed in the future will be explored, with reference to professional, statutory and regulatory requirements.

**interprofessional learning**
Occurs when two or more professions learn about, from and with each other, to enable effective collaboration and improve health outcomes.

## WHAT ARE THE DRIVERS FOR INTERPROFESSIONAL LEARNING?

The drivers for interprofessional learning mirror those for interprofessional working:

1 The voice of the patient
2 Policies and initiatives
3 Poor collaborative practice
4 Professional developments
5 Technological developments

In Chapter 2 we discussed these drivers with particular reference to inter-professional education. In this section we will focus on the UK health and social care policies and initiatives and the impact that regulatory bodies have had on the development of interprofessional learning.

## Policies and initiatives

The findings of public inquiries into the deaths of children have significantly influenced the developments in the education and training of all health and social care professionals.

Box 6.1 details the recommendations following these high-profile cases.

As can be seen from the recommendations, all these inquiries identified the need for more effective interprofessional education and training to promote collaborative working focused on the patient. Over the last 15 years the Department of Health has responded to recommendations from inquiries with the publication of a number of White Papers. These White Papers have shaped the current way in which health and social care professionals are educated both at undergraduate and post registration levels.

## BOX 6.1

**Learning from Bristol (Secretary of State for Health, 2001)**
This report into children's heart surgery at Bristol Royal Infirmary had among its 200 recommendations the following:

**Recommendation 57**
Greater priority than at present should be given to non-clinical aspects of care in six key areas in the education, training and continuing professional development of health care professionals:

- Skills in communicating with patients and with colleagues
- Education about the principles and organization of the NHS and about how care is managed, and the skills required for management
- The development of teamwork
- Shared learning across professional boundaries

- Clinical audit and reflective practice
- Leadership.

**Recommendation 61**
The education, training and continuing professional development (CPD) of all health care professionals should include joint courses between the professions.

**Recommendation 62**
There should be more opportunities than at present for multiprofessional teams to learn, train and develop together.

**Victoria Climbié Report (Secretary of State for Health, 2003)**
Similarly, the report into the death of Victoria Climbié had among its recommendations the following:

**Recommendation 14**
Each of the training bodies covering services provided by doctors, nurses, teachers, police officers, officers working in housing depart-

ments and social workers to demonstrate that effective joint working between each of these professional groups features in their national programmes.

**The Protection of Children in England: A Progress Report (Laming, 2009)**
**Recommendation 30**
All Children's Trusts should have multi-agency training to create a shared language and understanding of local referral procedures, assessment, information sharing and decision making across early years, schools, youth services, health, police and other services who work to protect children. A named child protection lead in each setting should receive this training.

**Recommendation 30**
The Department of Health should also take further steps to raise the profile and level of expertise for child protection within GP practices, for example by working with the Department for Children, Schools and Families to support joint training opportunities for GPs and children's social workers.

Although the inquiries into the deaths of children undergoing heart surgery at the Bristol Royal Infirmary and the deaths of Victoria Climbié and Baby Peter were set up in response to very different service failures, both reports had a consistent theme; the extent to which traditional divisions and demarcations between professions appeared to impede the need to work collaboratively in the interests of the patient.

## Making a Difference: Strengthening the Nursing, Midwifery and Health Visiting Contribution to Health and Health Care (Department of Health, 1999)

In this White Paper, the government outlined proposals to modernize education, training and regulation in nursing, midwifery and health visiting. This included providing more flexible career pathways into and within nursing; increasing the level of practical skills within the training programmes and delivering a nurse training system that was more responsive to the needs of the NHS. In the provision of continuing professional development (CPD), NHS organizations were to ensure that education programmes were focused on the development needs of clinical teams across traditional professional and service boundaries.

## The NHS Plan – A Plan for Investment, a Plan for Reform (Department of Health, 2000a)

This White Paper stressed the importance of collaboration between the NHS, higher education providers and regulatory bodies to make pre-registration training more flexible, with a core curriculum for common foundation programmes designed to promote partnership at all levels and to ensure seamless patient centred care. The core curriculum would include communications skills, and the NHS principles and organization. There was a clear commitment to providing pre-registration interprofessional education programmes for health and social care professionals with programmes that would promote teamwork, partnership and collaboration between professions.

## Meeting the Challenge: A Strategy for the Allied Health Professions (Department of Health, 2000b)

This White Paper outlined how education, training and regulation were to be modernized within the allied health professions and was based on the same general principles for modernizing the education, training and regulation for nurses, midwives and health visitors (Department of Health, 1999). Proposals outlined in this White Paper included more:

- flexible pathways into and through pre-registration programmes with opportunities to step on and off
- part-time programmes
- opportunities for shared learning
- innovative approaches to practice and fieldwork placements.

## A Health Service of all the Talents: Developing the NHS Workforce (Department of Health, 2000c)

In this White Paper, the government again confirmed its commitment to develop education and training arrangements which were 'genuinely' multiprofessional and which would enable students to transfer easily between courses without having to start their training from the beginning again.

## Working Together, Learning Together: A Framework for Lifelong Learning for the NHS (Department of Health, 2001)

This White Paper stated that all universities in England offering pre-registration professional education programmes should include common learning by 2004. Part of the government's commitment to the implementation of common learning was the funding of four 'leading-edge' sites. In 2002, the four leading-edge sites were announced. They were the higher education institutions at Newcastle; Kings College, London; Sheffield Hallam; and Southampton (Department of Health, 2002). These leading-edge sites had a broad remit which included to:

- develop common-learning programmes and core curricula for all professional staff in communications and NHS principles
- change workforce practices
- develop new ways of working
- break down professional and organizational barriers to learning and working together through closer integration of health professional programmes.

### The Knowledge and Skills Framework (NHS KSF) and the Development Review Process (Department of Health 2004a)

The Knowledge and Skills Framework was designed to support personal development in post, career development and service development, as well as to ensure transferability of roles, for all types and grades of NHS staff. The intention of this White Paper was to facilitate interprofessional working and therefore it had implications for interprofessional education (Barr *et al.*, 2011).

### The NHS Improvement Plan: Putting People at the Heart of Public Services (Department of Health (2004b)

This White Paper stated:

> Modernizing education, training and opportunities for learning are essential ... The Department has already funded joint programmes in common learning and interprofessional education between higher education and the NHS. These programmes will achieve national coverage as we ensure that people learn together so they may better work together in the NHS.
>
> Department of Health (2004b, p. 60)

### Creating an Interprofessional Workforce: An Education and Training Framework for Health and Social Care in England (Department of Health, 2007)

The Creating an Interprofessional Workforce (CIPW) project was funded by the Department of Health and the project team worked closely with the Centre for the Advancement of Interprofessional Education (CAIPE). The aim of the project was to produce an education and training framework for health and social care in England, which would support the development of an interprofessional workforce.

The Creating an Interprofessional Workforce project encompassed all educational levels within health and social care including pre-registration, post-registration education, practice based learning and development and informal learning in the workplace and the home through other activities such as volunteering.

The Report made recommendations to commissioners, education providers, employers and professional bodies.

### High Quality Workforce: NHS Next Stage Review (Department of Health, 2008)

This White Paper defines how the quality of care provided for patients will be enhanced through the NHS, Higher Education sector and industry working together to improve the quality of education and training offered in the NHS. This document addresses needs across the whole of the NHS workforce and links to social care, recognizing that teams work increasingly with others, particularly social care workers.

As can be seen, since 1999 when the White Paper *Making a Difference* (Department of Health, 1999) was published, there have been a number of significant White Papers which have shaped the education and training of health and social care professionals as we have moved into the 21st century. In this section, only key health and social care education and training policies have been discussed. There have, however, been other policies published which relate to specific service provision, for example, child health (Department for Education and Skills, 2005) and specific professions, for example, social work (Sharland *et al.*, 2007).

## Regulatory Bodies

Regulatory Bodies are now supporting pre-registration health and social care programmes to include interprofessional learning. For example, the Standards for Pre-registration Nursing Education in NMC state:

> ❝ *Programme providers must ensure that students have the opportunity to learn with, and from, other health and social care professionals.*
>
> NMC (2010, p. 75)

Whilst the Standards for Education and Training from the HPC state:

> ❝ *Successful interprofessional learning can develop students' ability to communicate and work with other professionals, potentially improving the environment for service users and professionals.*
>
> HPC (2009, p. 40)

For social work the Department of Health requires providers to:

> ❝ *Demonstrate that all students undertake specific learning and assessment in partnership working and information sharing across professional disciplines and agencies.*
>
> Department of Health (2002, p. 4)

The General Medical Council (GMC) state:

> ❝ *Medical schools must ensure that students work with and learn from other health and social care professionals and students.*
>
> GMC (2009, p. 52)

As we can see from this discussion, government polices and Regulatory Bodies are ensuring that interprofessional education does happen. This should result in effective interprofessional collaboration within the practice setting and the consequent enhancement of the quality of care provided to patients.

# LEARNING THEORIES AND INTERPROFESSIONAL EDUCATION

Learning undertaken by health and social care professionals in the practice setting can take many forms and is affected by the working environment and practice activity. Therefore, there are a range of learning theories that can contribute to understanding and implementing interprofessional education within the practice setting (Hean *et al.*, 2012; Hean and Craddock, 2009; Reeves *et al.*, 2007).

These learning theories broadly fall into two categories:

1 Those that focus on the individual, for example, constructivist and behaviourist approaches.

2 Those that view learning as a collective process, for example, social constructivism.

Whilst one type of learning theory will not inform all practice contexts, in this section we will consider two social constructivist theories: activity theory and situated learning theory.

Health and social care in the 21st century emphasizes the benefits of interprofessional working, systems-based patient safety and organizational learning (Bleakley, 2006). Therefore, health and social care takes place within a complex system which is comprised of many components that are dynamic and continuously interact, including: multiplicity of interactions and relationships among individual learners and practitioners; teams; education and health systems and organizations; environments and cultures. All of these factors influence what is learned and what is applied in practice (D'Amour and Oandasan, 2005).

Social constructivist models of learning take into account all these factors and these theories, therefore, seem suited to interprofessional education.

## What is activity theory?

Engeström (2001) is the central theorist in the field of activity theory. In this theory the learner is not simply socialized into the knowledge held by the community or activity in a passive manner. The learner's participation acts as a disturbance to an already unstable system that offers collaborative knowledge production over a period of time (Bleakley, 2006).

Engeström's work (2001) focuses on work based learning within the health care setting within six specific related activity systems. The relationship between these six activity systems can be seen in Figure 6.1.

1 **Object**
   Every system has an object or focus of interest, for health and social care practitioners this would be the patient.

2 **Subject**
   The subject is the people engaged in the activities, for example, the health or social care practitioners engaged in the care of the patient.

3 **Community or community of practice**
This is the social context, so this might be the ward team providing the care for the patient.

4 **Tools or artefacts**
Tools are influenced by culture, and their use is a way for the accumulation and transmission of social knowledge. Examples of tools or artefacts within health and social care include: professional language; clinical images, investigation results.

5 **Roles/divisions of labour**
This is the division of activities amongst those in the system. For example, within a ward team this might be the medical staff, nurses, occupational therapists, physiotherapists.

6 **Rules**
Rules are the conventions, guidelines and rules that regulate activities in the system, for example, hand washing protocols, health and safety policies.

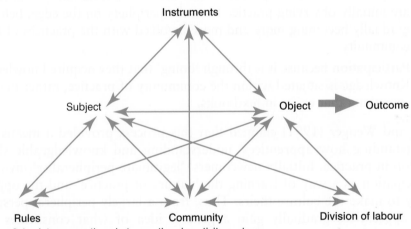

Figure 6.1   Interconnections between the six activity systems

It is the relationship between and within each activity system that makes this learning theory ideal to use in interprofessional education. This model of learning tells us how new knowledge is produced and held collaboratively in inherently unstable, complex systems such as those found in health and social care.

## What is situated learning?

This exploration of situated learning will be based on the work of Lave (1988) and Lave and Wenger (1991). Lave and Wenger are key proponents in the field of situated learning.

Lave and Wenger's (1991) theory of situated learning evolved from the historical forms of apprenticeship, whereby students spent a considerable period of time, usually five years, learning their craft from a 'master'. This form of training focuses on the gradual acquisition of craft knowledge through demonstration and practice, with feedback. Until recently, learning through apprenticeship was assumed to be concrete, context-embedded, intuitive, limited in scope of its application, mechanical, rote, imitative, not creative, and out of date. However, recently there has been renewed interest in situated learning as a model of how professionals learn to apply practical knowledge within infinitely varied social contexts. Central to Lave and Wenger's theory is a process called 'legitimate peripheral participation'. This is a rather complex term and can be best understood by considering the three components of this phrase separately. All three components depend on each other:

1 It is **legitimate** because everyone involved accepts the position of learners/new team members/newly qualified practitioners as potential members of the community of practice.

2 **Peripheral** because the 'potential' members of the community of practice are initially observing practice from the periphery on the edge, before gradually becoming more and more involved with the practices of the community.

3 **Participation** because it is through 'doing' that they acquire knowledge. Knowledge is situated within the community of practice, rather than something that exists in textbooks.

Lave and Wenger (1991) claimed that this process provided a means for understanding how apprentices' understanding and knowledgeable skills develop in practice. Initially newcomers' 'legitimate peripherality' involves participation as a way of learning the 'culture of practice' and the opportunity to make the culture theirs. Thus, from a largely peripheral perspective, apprentices gradually gain a general idea of what constitutes the practice of the community. Over a period of time, the newcomers' understanding of old-timers increases, for example newcomers know how, when and about what old-timers collaborate, disagree/agree about and what they enjoy, dislike, respect and admire. The process of 'legitimate peripheral participation' (Figure 6.2) provides the newcomers with exemplars as they move towards full participation in the community of practice. Partial participation is a dynamic process in which the newcomer can gain access to sources of understanding through growing involvement in the community of practice.

Lave and Wenger's (1991) theory moves the focus of learning away from the individual towards the community, emphasizing the view that learning is an integral and inseparable aspect of social practice.

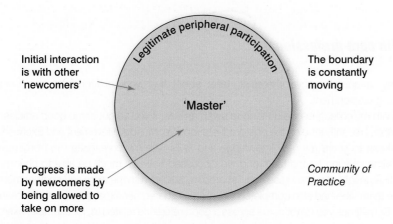

Figure 6.2   Diagram to illustrate 'legitimate peripheral participation'
Note this diagram is not endorsed by Lave and Wenger (1991) and is purely representational

The key features of a community of practice are:

● Communities of practice are everywhere – at home, at work, at university. We all belong to a number of them.

● Communities of practice are informally bound by what they do together and by what they have learned through their mutual engagement in these activities.

● Communities of practice develop around things that matter to people.

● The practices of a community reflect the members' own understanding of what is important.

● Communities of practice are defined by what the community is about; how it functions and what capability it has produced.

## Reflective activity

Think of a community of practice that you have been involved in as a 'newcomer' and consider the following:

● Who was involved in the community of practice?

● Draw a diagram to show who you interacted with and who interacted with you.

● Who did you respect and why?

● What did the long-standing members enjoy about working within the community of practice?

● What did the long-standing members debate/discuss/disagree with each other about?

● Think about how well the community of practice functioned as a team.

*Health care professional*

Hayley, a qualified physiotherapist, talks about her work environment also being a learning environment.

"With my colleagues we do tend to swap articles, if you've got some good articles. For example, I recently studied the postgraduate module, Muscle, Movement and Exercise and was keen to share my new knowledge and skills with my colleagues. So I organized a lunchtime meeting for the team and we discussed how we might be able to change our practices in light of current research. I shared my articles with the team and another member of the team who had also completed this module shared her experiences with the team as well. Sometimes you might come across a good reference related to, for example, exercise, or they give it to you and you are then able to look it up, so yes, we do share tips, our knowledge, to improve our professional knowledge and enhance our patient care."

## KEY POINTS

- Situated learning theory recognizes that knowledge is embedded within the context in which it is used and cannot be separated from the activity, context and culture of that situation

- Learners engage in situated learning by negotiating meaning with one another through the use of tools and artefacts such as language, books, music and art

- Learning takes place as a result of participating in 'real' activities that nurture and guide the learner's ability to think

- Learners develop a shared understanding about the purpose of the community and develop a sense of belonging

## EVIDENCE BASE

To read a critique of activity theory and situated learning theory locate and read this article:

- Arnseth, H.C. (2008) Activity theory and situated learning theory: contrasting views of educational practice. *Pedagogy, Culture & Society,* **16**(3): 289–302.

## CREATING AN INTERPROFESSIONAL LEARNING ENVIRONMENT

We will now consider the specific approaches toward learning and teaching which a community of practice could embrace to create an interprofessional learning environment. These features centre on fostering varied learning and teaching strategies that encourage the newcomers and old-timers of a community of practice to develop both personally and professionally. These learning and teaching strategies include frameworks for learning (for example, critical appreciation, cooperative learning, collaboration, coaching) and tools for learning (for example reflection, narratives). We will discuss these frameworks and tools below.

## Frameworks for learning

### Critical appreciation

Critical appreciation, a term that comes from the arts, is a process to enable practitioners to express their insights into professional practice. It is concerned with recognizing, in a sensitive and holistic way, the qualities of practice and thinking critically about the values, traditions, beliefs and assumptions that underlie its surface (Fish, 1989). It involves the practitioners themselves investigating their own work but as part of their normal duties. A key activity in critical appreciation is for practitioners to bring the personal professional knowledge embedded in their practice to the surface and to consider it critically in the light of the context, the traditions and conventions of their profession as a whole.

Critical appreciation is not unproblematic, because for many health and social care professions, particularly scientific-based professions, the idea of conceptualizing practice as art and seeing their work as artistry, is an alien concept. Therefore, initially, a great deal of time would need to be invested by the members of a community to help both newcomers and old-timers to develop the skills and language that are necessary for artistic writing. Also, the success of professional artistry relies on the practitioner not only being willing to see practice anew but to deliberately look at practice from a different viewpoint.

Critical appreciation also requires practitioners to develop their self-critical skills, to enable them to gain self-knowledge regarding their performance. These skills are difficult to acquire and self-comment often tends to be justificatory rather than critical.

### Cooperative learning

Cooperative learning is very effective in promoting learning to work in teams (Shimazoe and Aldrich, 2010). This makes cooperative learning an essential framework for inclusion within an interprofessional learning environment.

Healthy cooperative learning has five important and necessary features (Johnson and Johnson, 2009):

1 **Positive interdependence**
   Positive interdependence means being interconnected. Learners strive together to reach a common goal, with each learner's efforts being required and indispensable to the group's success. The learners 'sink or swim together' and there can be no 'free riders'. Each group member has a

unique contribution to make to the joint effort because of their resources and/or role and task responsibilities. Group members provide mutual support and encouragement and celebrate their joint success together.

An example of a common goal would be the completion of a task such as a patient problem that required a range of health and social professionals to work together to make a joint decision.

2 **Face-to-face promotive interaction**
Promotive interaction can be defined as individuals encouraging and facilitating each other's efforts to achieve, complete tasks and produce in order to reach the group's goals. This is usually synchronous, purposeful activity such as discussion, debate and joint decision making.

3 **Individual accountability**
Individual accountability means that each individual is assessed for mastery of the content of a task and is held responsible for contributing a fair share to the success of the group. This is an important factor because it means that no one can opt out of learning or be allowed to hide behind the work of others.

4 **Interpersonal and small-group skills**
This involves teaching members of the team skills needed to succeed. In order for learners to coordinate efforts to achieve mutual goals, learners must get to know and trust each other, communicate accurately and unambiguously, accept and support each other, and resolve conflict constructively.

5 **Group processing**
Group processing is reflecting on the actions, both group and individual, to describe what actions were helpful and unhelpful and to make decisions about what actions to continue or change. The purpose of group processing is to clarify and improve the effectiveness of the members contributing to the collaboration efforts in order to achieve the group goals.

These five essential elements of cooperative learning promote both interprofessional teamwork and interprofessional learning within the practice environment.

## Reflective activity

Think of a learning activity that is focused on providing optimal care for the patient within an interprofessional environment. Using the five essential elements of the cooperative learning model consider the following:

1  What is the common goal for the learning activity?

2  Who are the members of the interprofessional team involved in achieving the common goal?

3  What methods will be used to encourage face-to-face promotive interaction?

4 How will the individual group members and the team be assessed for their mastery of skills and contribution to the team activity?

5 How will you facilitate the development of team skills?

6 What methods will you use in the team activity to facilitate reflection on the effectiveness of the team in achieving its goals?

## Collaboration

Collaboration between old-timers and newcomers within a community of practice is a key concept of situated learning. Vygotsky (1978), a Russian psychologist, identified a 'zone of proximal development' in which a learner's development occurs through participation in activities slightly beyond their competence with the assistance of more skilled practitioners. Learning takes place in the zone of proximal development via interactions between an individual's personal knowledge system and the social knowledge system.

## Coaching

Coaching, another key aspect of an interprofessional learning environment, is centred on unlocking a practitioner's potential to maximize their own performance. It models many aspects of interprofessional working, enabling health and social care professionals to learn about each other as they learn together.

Coaching is an ideal framework for learning as it has the adaptability to support different practitioners with different learning styles within the community of practice. A coaching relationship is one of collaboration, with the emphasis being on enabling the practitioner to fully develop their skills and to facilitate a shift in their knowledge and behaviour. Key elements of coaching include: identification of specific goals; focused learning opportunities and challenges; provision of feedback; time for reflection, analysis and action planning; and support.

Within a community of practice, coaching provides a flexible development approach for individual practitioners that can be delivered at the right time and in parallel with the community's need to constantly change and adapt to an ever-changing environment.

## EVIDENCE BASE

Read the following article: Locke, A. (2008) Developmental Coaching: Bridge to Organizational Success. *Creative Nursing*, **14**(3): 102–110.

This article discusses the relevance of developmental coaching and provides examples of its potential within the health care setting.

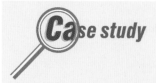

## Coaching for career development

Paul is a senior staff nurse working in the accident and emergency (A&E) department of a large teaching hospital. He is unsure as to whether or not he wishes to stay working as a clinical nurse or whether to look at other opportunities to further his career. As part of Paul's professional development plan he is offered the opportunity of having a coach who is external to his organization. Paul takes up this opportunity and has now met three times with his coach, Alison. Alison is an effective coach who listens, discusses and questions what Paul is saying to try and clarify Paul's sense of purpose, core values and beliefs. She helps Paul to clarify his vision for his future and explore whether this is a reality, whilst at the same time providing encouragement and motivation to improve his confidence. Alison provides Paul with the support, some ideas, know-how and tools to help him make a decision. Paul, with the support of Alison, decides to explore the possibility of pursuing a career in nurse education. Alison has helped Paul reach this decision through effective listening and questioning and encouraging him to explore his own values, drivers, commitment and purpose and whether these align to a career in education.

Paul is really pleased with the opportunity provided by his current employer to help him consider the future direction of his career. He considered one of the most valuable aspects of the coaching was the 'me time' that it provided, and the opportunity to have this time to explore this with someone from outside of the organization.

### *Reflection*

Reflective practice is associated with learning from experience and as such is a key learning and teaching strategy within a situated-learning environment. Using the process of reflection within a community of practice will help to generate practice-based knowledge and offers a practice-based learning activity that not only contributes to the continuing professional development (CPD) of the individual practitioner but also to the continuing development of the community.

Reflection within the health and social care setting is a prerequisite to professional caring. It is an intentional activity that enables the practitioner to become more self-aware of the contradictions that exist between how we would like to practise and how we actually do. Engaging in reflective practice is associated with improving and changing practice and stimulating personal and professional growth.

Johns defines reflection as:

> ❝ *Being mindful of self, either within or after experience, as if a mirror in which the practitioner can view and focus self within the context of a particular experience, in order to confront, understand and move toward resolving contradiction between one's vision and actual practice.*

*Johns (2009)*

When we, as health and social care practitioners think of reflection, how do we perceive it? In one sense, reflection relates to the carrying out of a number of practices and our understanding of them; in another it relates to thoughts, feelings and understanding of particular events. But how well do we reflect, how well do we use reflection and how does the reflective process sit within a situated-learning environment?

The work of Donald Schon is widely regarded as the most seminal on the subject of reflection in professional practice. Schon (1983) identifies two types of reflection: reflection-in-action and reflection-on-action. Reflection-in-action is the process whereby the practitioner recognizes a new situation or a problem and thinks about it while still acting. Reflection-on-action, on the other hand, is the retrospective contemplation of practice undertaken in order to uncover knowledge used in a particular situation, by analysing and interpreting the information recalled.

There have been a number of structured models of reflection developed to encourage practitioners to reflect on their practice, including Gibbs (1998); Atkins and Murphy (1993); Johns (2006) and Driscoll (2000).

## Reflective activity

Look up the models of reflection mentioned in the last paragraph and consider which one(s) you feel would provide the most appropriate strategy to guide your reflection.

The use of structured reflection models fosters a mechanistic approach towards reflection. This may result in reflection becoming cold, detached and devoid of the nature of caring, representative of technical processes as opposed to dynamic relationships, and lacking in the real representation of skilled health and social care practice.

If practitioners viewed their work as art, reflections on both their *practices* and *thoughts* on practice could be represented through the symbolism of art. Practitioners could look deep into their portrait of practice, considering, for example, its composition, tone, subject matter, space and form. These concepts are taken from the arts and used when critically analyzing paintings (Acton, 1997). Using these concepts to reflect on practice can lead practitioners through uncovering layers of knowledge and practice, revealing the meaning of the practices, or enabling practitioners to apply layers to the existing professional practice. Practitioners' portraits of practice can be represented, for example, as stories, paintings, mime and poetry (Law, 2011).

This approach to reflection would enable learners to develop an appreciation of the complexities of their practice and that of their community of practice.

## Narratives

Narratives, when used as part of a learning and teaching strategy, can be of considerable value in both the personal and professional development of health and social care practitioners.

Health and social care practitioners know patients through the stories patients tell and health and social care practitioners respond with stories of their own. The knowledge the practitioner gains about a patient is extended into further narratives when conveyed to others. Stories are told about stories and narratives thus become a form of social interaction.

Narrative provides meaning, context and perspective for health and social care practice. It is a way of knowing – a discovery – which defines how, why and in what way practice is occurring. Narrative offers practitioners a possibility of understanding that cannot be arrived at by any other means. Narratives are a way in which the individual can gain personal knowledge and social knowledge, offering a learning opportunity which gives the individual the freedom to be who they are, rather than comply with the practitioner's vision of optimal practice. Biases, assumptions and prejudices are encountered so that new possibilities for connection are discovered. The use of narrative as a learning strategy to promote the humanistic dimensions of care has been used in medicine (Greenhalgh and Hurwitz, 1998), nursing (Benner et al., 1996), physiotherapy (Jenson et al., 1999) and social work (Balen et al., 2009). Narratives are undoubtedly a learning strategy that could be used by all health and social care professions. As Greenhalgh and Hurwitz succinctly state:

In the education of patients and professionals, narratives:

- are often memorable
- are grounded in experience
- enforce reflection.

*Greenhalgh and Hurwitz (1998, p. 7)*

What is a narrative?

- It has a beginning, middle and end.
- It has a narrator and a listener and is thereby created in a relationship.
- The narrative is concerned with the individual.
- The choice of what to tell and what to omit lies entirely with the narrator.
- It engages the listener and invites an interpretation.
- It is a means of developing professional knowledge.

Stories have the potential to reveal what is significant and relevant to the practitioners about situations and events in their practice. Providing the practitioner with the occasion to tell their story and also to hear their story affords the practitioner the opportunity to reflect upon the paths and options that they did not take at the time and perhaps consider ones that did not occur when the event took place.

## Reflective activity

Select a practice skill that a learner you are working with needs to acquire.

Use the situated learning model to design and develop a learning environment that is suitable for the learner to acquire the practice skill. Consider the following:

- Think about which members of the community of practice will be involved in facilitating the development of the practice skill.
- Consider where in the community of practice the learning should take place.
- What learning and teaching strategies will you use and why?
- Think about the role that you will adopt within the situated activity.

## KEY POINTS

The key points of a situated-learning environment are:

- that it fosters the development of lifelong learning skills
- that situated learning and teaching strategies include critical appreciation; cooperative learning; collaboration; reflection; coaching and narrative
- that learning takes place in the zone of proximal development through interactions between a newcomer and an old-timer
- that the learner and the facilitator are actively involved in and jointly manage the responsibility for learning
- situated learning techniques take more time and effort for both the learner and facilitator.

## SUPPORTING LEARNERS IN THE PRACTICE ENVIRONMENT

It is essential that learners are supported within the practice environment to enable them to develop both personally and professionally. In the health and social care professions, this support is usually provided by a professional who takes on the role of a mentor. A mentor may also be described as a supervisor, facilitator, clinical supervisor, practice teacher, clinical lecturer or placement educator. In this section, the term 'mentor' (and the related 'mentorship') encompasses all these terms.

In 2000 the Department of Health document *Meeting the Challenge: A Strategy for the Allied Health Professionals* (Department of Health, 2000b, p. 5) stated: 'supervising students is a key part of every professional practitioner's role'. Supervising students is now incorporated into a number of professional codes of conducts:

> ❝ *Nurses and midwives on the NMC professional register have a duty to 'facilitate students of nursing and midwifery and others to develop their competence'.*

*NMC (2008a, Standard 23)*

The British Medical Association (2004) emphasizes that mentoring should be available to all medical students for confidential, professional and personal advice.

Although these documents are written by specific professional bodies, the issues raised regarding the quality of mentorship and the role of the mentor are pertinent to all health and social care professions.

## History of mentoring

The term 'mentoring' originates in Greek mythology. The Greek poet Homer in his epic poem the *Odyssey* first used the word 'mentor'. In his poem, Homer tells the story of *Odysseus* who went away to fight the Trojan War leaving the care of his son Telemachus to his wise and trusted friend Mentor. The relationship between Mentor and Telemachus was described as nurturing, educative and protective. It ensured Telemachus's personal and social development and also that he was prepared professionally for his responsibilities and tasks ahead.

In more recent times, the idea of mentoring has attracted attention from trainers, educators, policy makers and the business world, all of them interested in initial and continuing professional development. Mentoring first became popular during the 1970s and 1980s as a method of professional development in the USA. In the late 1980s, the private sector in the UK began to take a keen interest in the potential of mentoring and in the 1990s mentoring began to cross the public–private divide.

Today, mentoring has been embraced by many diverse organizations and professions and has been described as 'a developmental alliance', occupying an important position in the initial and continuing development of many health and social care professionals.

## What is mentoring?

Mentoring has been variously defined within and outside of the health and social care professions, which has led to there being no agreement on the meaning of the term. Oxley, for example, defines mentoring as:

> ❝ *The process whereby an experienced, highly regarded, empathic person (the mentor), guides another individual (the mentee) in the development and re-examination of their own ideas, learning and personal and professional development. The mentor, who often, but*

*not necessarily, works in the same organization or field as the mentee, achieves this by listening and talking in confidence to the mentee.*

*Oxley (1998, cited in BMA, 2004, p. 3)*

Other definitions include Goppe (2011, p. 3) who has defined mentoring as helping an individual to learn during their developmental years, to progress towards and achieve maturity and establish their identity. Hayes (2005) defines mentorship as an intense relationship between a novice and an expert to promote role socialization and, ultimately, role success of the novice. Clutterbuck (2004) defines mentoring as principally listening with empathy, mutually sharing experiences, professional friendship, developing insight through reflection and being a sounding board.

These examples highlight that the term 'mentoring' means different things to different people and as a consequence there is no agreed definition. However, what all health and social professions have in common is the commitment to teach, support, coach, facilitate, assess and supervise students in practice, providing professional role modelling, to ensure that students are fit for purpose and practice.

In nursing and midwifery, there is a requirement that all nursing and midwifery students are assigned a mentor for the duration of their practice placement. To undertake the role of a mentor, nursing and midwifery practitioners must have undertaken a mentorship programme or equivalent, which is approved by the Nursing and Midwifery Council (NMC). In 2008 the NMC published the document 'Standards to support learning and assessment in practice' which identify eight domains which represent the competencies and outcomes for mentors. Each domain is broken down into several outcomes (See Box 6.2). In addition, to remain a mentor, mentors are required to attend and record an annual mentor update.

Similarly, for operating department practitioners (ODP) there is a requirement for mentors to have completed a recognized qualification prior to mentoring ODP students (CODP, 2009) and to attend and record an annual mentor update.

In other professions, for example, radiography, occupational therapy, physiotherapy, there is no requirement for mentors to have completed a recognized mentor qualification, but all professions have a strategy for ensuring that professionals who take on the role of mentor are appropriately trained and have annual mentor updates.

## BOX 6.2

### NMC (2008b) Mentor Domains

| | |
|---|---|
| 1 Establish effective working relationships | 5 Creating an environment for learning |
| 2 Facilitation of learning | 6 Context of practice |
| 3 Assessment and accountability | 7 Evidence-based practice |
| 4 Evaluation of learning | 8 Leadership |

## What is the role of a mentor?

Within the literature a mentor is defined by the various roles that the mentor undertakes. I would like to suggest the following definition for a mentor which encompasses all the roles: an experienced professional who teaches, supports, advises, guides, acts as a resource and role model and promotes self-development, fulfilment of potential and confidence in the learner (mentee) achieving both professional and life goals.

There is no single personality type that is synonymous with that of being or becoming an effective mentor. You can find, within the literature, an extensive range of characteristics or qualities which students consider to be essential in a good mentor. These have been listed in Table 6.1 under headings regarding the roles undertaken by a mentor. This list is by no means exhaustive and is not presented in any particular order.

| Table 6.1 Qualities students consider important in a mentor | |
| --- | --- |
| Personal qualities | • Enthusiastic, friendly, approachable<br>• Patient and understanding<br>• Sense of humour<br>• Non-judgemental, tolerant and accepts personal differences<br>• Trustworthy |
| Role model | • Organized<br>• Able to set a good example<br>• Confident and secure with self, cares about others and treats everyone with respect |
| Teacher | • Effective communicator<br>• Knowledgeable and up to date in their field<br>• Able to help with goal setting and planning<br>• Willing to share personal experiences, knowledge and skills<br>• Good source of information |
| Guide/supervisor | • Able to encourage personal and professional development<br>• Able to instil confidence and motivate people<br>• Proactive, imaginative and creative<br>• Open to other points of view<br>• Realistic expectations of the student<br>• Able to know when to give and when not to give advice<br>• Able to act as a friend while at the same time providing guidance |
| Assessor | • Prepared to use constructive criticism<br>• Provides regular feedback on the student's performance |

Mentors have a pivotal role to play in the delivery of the next generation of health and social care professionals. Those mentors involved in supporting pre-registration students have a responsibility to ensure that the student is fit for purpose, fit for practice and fit for award before the student gains their licence to practice from the appropriate regulatory body, for example the Nursing and Midwifery Council, or Health Professions Council. Mentors therefore act as gatekeepers to their profession and take responsibility for protecting the public.

## Health care professional

Naveen, an experienced community nurse and mentor, speaks of her experiences as a mentor.

"Although initially I felt that I had little choice in becoming a mentor, on reflection it has been a thoroughly worthwhile experience, although frustrating at times. The challenge has always been attempting to juggle patient needs, team management, course requirements and student expectations all at the same time! However, over the nine years of being a mentor within the community setting the rewards have much outweighed those difficulties.

The greatest satisfaction comes from students coming back to your area year on year as this enables you to see how they are progressing, not only in skills and competence, but also in self-belief that they can actually achieve their goal of becoming a registered nurse. Seeing staff nurses in the corridor in the local hospital who still remember you as their mentor, hopefully fondly, or students who had not thought of a community nursing career return to community nursing posts once qualified is fantastic. It's nice to think that maybe I, in some small way, might have made a difference to that student."

## EVIDENCE BASE

Read *Guide series: Mentoring Framework* (National Workforce Projects, NHS), which is a document providing information that will help you understand the process of mentoring and provides helpful tips on being a good mentor.

## Reflective activity

Think about a health- or social-care practitioner who has been your mentor. Consider the following:

- What do you feel were the strengths and weaknesses of your mentor?
- How did your mentor's strengths and weaknesses influence the quality of your learning experience while you were assigned to your mentor?
- As a learner, how could you have improved this mentor–learner relationship?

## INTERPROFESSIONAL MENTORSHIP

As we have seen, mentorship has a long history, but the concept of inter-professional mentorship is relatively new and in its infancy in health and social care professions. It is essential that learners are supported appropriately within interprofessional situated-learning environments. Interprofessional mentorship would appear to be the way ahead for supporting learners and this is now being supported by a number of the Professional, Statutory and Regulatory Bodies. For example the CODP (2009, p. 26) have articulated the value of interprofessional mentoring and how this may take place within the practice setting. Also the CODP have stated that the mentor must:

> ❝ Demonstrate an understanding of interprofessional issues in practice and how this impacts on learning, and how this learning can be facilitated in practice.

> *CODP (2009, p. 17)*

For nurses and midwives the following reference is made to interprofessional working within the NMC Standards for mentors, practice teachers and teachers:

> ❝ Demonstrate effective relationship building skills sufficient to support learning as part of a wider interprofessional team for a range of students in both practice and academic learning environments.

> *NMC (2008b p. 62)*

## What is interprofessional mentorship?

At the current time, there is a dearth of literature relating to interprofessional mentorship, only Marshall and Gordon (2005, 2010) and Lait *et al.* (2011) have published in this area. Marshall and Gordon define interprofessional mentorship as:

> ❝ Occasions when a health or social care professional facilitates interprofessional learning and supervises and assesses students in the practice setting.

> *Marshall and Gordon (2005, p. 39)*

Whereas Lait *et al.* define interprofessional mentorship as:

> ❝ Learning that takes place between providers and students who are from different disciplines or health professions.

> *Lait* et al. *(2011, p. 211)*

The focus of interprofessional mentorship, therefore, is to facilitate learning opportunities for students to enable them to learn from and with professionals from their own and other professions in the practice setting. The patient is always at the centre of the interprofessional learning experience, with the overall aim being to improve collaboration between different professional groups and the quality of care. Thus, interprofessional mentorship will focus on the facilitation of the knowledge, skills and understanding required to work successfully within the interprofessional context.

## The key characteristics of an interprofessional mentor?

Earlier in this chapter we identified the key characteristics of a mentor, which included effective communication and interpersonal skills, being enthusiastic, friendly, approachable, organized, patient, understanding, caring, knowledgeable and up to date in their field, able to help with goal setting and planning, and acting as a good source of information (see Table 6.1).

If we review these key characteristics of a uniprofessional mentor, it can be seen that these are generic rather than profession-specific skills. It would therefore be possible for mentors to transfer these skills to situations involving learners from different professional groups. The one skill relevant to interprofessional mentorship that cannot be transferred is that of profession specific knowledge. However, Marshall and Gordon (2010, p. 363) consider that the central focus of interprofessional mentorship is interprofessional learning and working and it is this aspect of knowledge that should be considered for successful interprofessional mentorship. This would make interprofessional mentorship a possibility for all mentors and all learners, regardless of the professional background.

## EVIDENCE BASE

Read the following article, Marshall, M. and Gordon, F. (2010) Exploring the role of the interprofessional mentor. *Journal of Interprofessional Care,* **24**(4): 362–374.

This article discusses a model for interprofessional mentorship, which has been developed from qualitative interviews with students and health and social care professionals who support students in practice settings.

Read the Deutshlander, S. and Suter. E. (2011) *Interprofessional Mentoring Guide.* Canada: Alberta Health Services. This is available from: http://www.albertahealthservices. ca/careers/docs/WhereDoYouFit/wduf-stu-sp-ip-mentoring-guide.pdf

Although this is a Canadian publication it offers a comprehensive guide to interprofessional mentoring for mentors and students which is equally applicable in the UK and other countries.

# What is the role of an interprofessional mentor?

The primary roles of an interprofessional mentor are the same as those of a uniprofessional mentor, that is, the facilitation of learning, supervision and assessment of learners in the practice environment. The application of these roles, however, would be related to the learner's interprofessional learning outcomes.

As we discussed earlier in this chapter, learners currently have profession-specific interprofessional learning outcomes articulated, as well as profession-specific learning outcomes. The Interprofessional Capability Framework (CUILU, 2004) and revised six years later (Sheffield Hallam University, 2010) was developed to offer interprofessional learning outcomes that were applicable to all health and social care learners.

The Interprofessional Capability Framework offers a way of describing what any undergraduate student of health- or social care needs to learn to work collaboratively. The framework has been divided into four domains: collaborative working, reflection, cultural awareness and ethical practice, and organizational competence. Each domain contains three levels of learning that lead incrementally to achieving the capability.

The framework provides those involved in delivering interprofessional education with a tool for identifying approaches to collaborative learning and working within the university setting and, importantly, within a range of practice contexts. In addition, the framework can provide a focus for the assessment of capabilities that might be met by a learner spending time with a practitioner from another profession.

Canada has also published Interprofessional Competency Framework (CIHC, 2010) that guides interprofessional education and collaborative practice for all professions in a variety of contexts. This framework has six domains: role clarification, patient/client/family/community-centred care, team functioning, collaborative leadership, interprofessional communication and interprofessional conflict resolution. These six domains emphasize the knowledge, skills, attitudes and values that are essential for interprofessional collaborative practice.

It is interesting to note the use of the word capability in the title of English framework and competency in the Canadian framework. The word capability has been used in the English framework because it suggests, rather than an end point of learning, that of becoming competent, that development is ongoing and there is a continuation of learning (Sheffield Hallam University, 2010, p. 5). Whereas competency has been used in the Canadian framework to enable the learner to master those situations they will have to deal with in their professional and/or private life (CIHC, 2010, p. 7).

## *Reflective activity*

Read the Interprofessional Capability Framework (Sheffield Hallam, 2010). This document is available from: **http://www.hsaparchive.org.uk/doc/resources/icf2010.pdf/at_download/file.pdf**

Read the National Interprofessional Competency Framework (CIHC, 2010). This document is available from: **http://www.cihc.ca/files/CIHC_IPCompetencies_Feb1210.pdf**

When you have read the two frameworks select one domain from each framework and consider the following:

1 Do you have the necessary knowledge, skills, attitudes and values to demonstrate that meet the level expected within the selected domains?

2 If you feel that there are aspects of the domains that you need to further develop, write an action plan to show how you are going to achieve the requirements of the domains.

3 Discuss your action plan with your mentor when you are next in the practice setting.

## RAPID RECAP

Check your progress so far by working through each of the following questions.

1 What are the key features of a community of practice?

2 List the key points of situated learning theory.

3 What are the key features of a situated-learning environment?

4 What is the role of an interprofessional mentor?

If you have difficulty with more than one of the questions, read through the section again to refresh your understanding before moving on.

# REFERENCES

Acton, M. (1997) *Learning to look at paintings.* London: Routledge.

Atkins, S. and Murphy, K. (1993) Reflection: a review of the literature. *Journal of Advanced Nursing,* 18(8): 1188–1192.

Balen, R., Rhodes, C., and Ward, L. (2009) The power of stories: using narrative for interdisciplinary learning in Health and Social Care. *Social Work Education: The International Journal,* 29(4): 416–426.

Barr, H., Koppel, I., Reeves, S., Hammick, M. and Freeth, D. (2005) *Effective interprofessional education: assumption, argument and evidence.* London: Blackwell.

Benner, P., Tanner, C.A. and Chesla, C.A. (1996) *Expertise in nursing practice.* New York: Springer.

Bleakley, A. (2006) Broadening conceptions of learning in medical education: The message from teamworking. *Medical Education,* 40: 150–157.

British Medical Association (2004) *Exploring mentoring.* BMA, London. Available from: www.bma.org.uk/ap.nsf/Content/Mentoring/$file/mentoring.pdf.

Brookfield, S. (2009) The concept of critical reflection: promises and contradictions. *European Journal of Social Work,* 12(3): 293–304.

Canadian Interprofessional Health Collaborative (2010) A national interprofessional competency framework. Available from: http://www.cihc.ca/files/CIHC_IPCompetencies_Feb1210.pdf. Accessed July 2012.

Clutterbuck, D. (2004) *Everybody needs a mentor.* London: Chartered Institute of Personnel Development.

College of Operating Department Practitioners (2009) *Standards, recommendations and guidance for mentors and practice placements.* London: CODP.

Cooper, H., Carlisle, C., Gibbs, T. and Watkins, C. (2001) Developing an evidence base for interdisciplinary learning: A systematic literature review. *Journal of Advanced Nursing,* 35(2): 228–237.

CUILU (2004) *The Interprofessional Capability Framework.* Available from: http://www.cuilu.group.shef.ac.uk/capability_framework.pdf. Accessed July 2012.

D'Amour, D. and Oandasan, I. (2005) Interprofessionality as the field of interprofessional practice and interprofessional education: an emerging concept. *Journal of Interprofessional Care,* 19 Suppl 1: 8–20.

Department of Health (1999) *Making a difference: strengthening the nursing, midwifery and health visiting contribution to health and health care.* London: Department of Health.

Department of Health (2000a) *The NHS Plan: a plan for investment, a plan for reform.* London: Department of Health.

Department of Health (2000b) *Meeting the challenge: a strategy for the allied health professions.* London: Department of Health.

Department of Health (2000c) *A health service of all the talents: developing the NHS workforce.* London: Department of Health.

Department of Health (2001) *Working together, learning together: a framework for lifelong learning for the NHS.* London: Department of Health.

Department of Health (2002) *Requirements for social work training.* London: Department of Health.

Department of Health (2004a) *The knowledge and skills framework (NHS KSF) and the development review process.* London: Department of Health.

Department of Health (2004b) *The NHS improvement plan: putting people at the heart of public services.* London: Department of Health.

Department of Health (2007) *Creating an interprofessional workforce: an education and training framework for health and social care in England.* London: Department of Health.

Department of Health (2008) *High quality workforce: NHS next stage review.* London: HMSO.

Department for Education and Skills (2005) *Common core skills and knowledge for the children's workforce.* London: DfES Publications.

Deutshlander, S. and Suter, E. (2011) *Interprofessional mentoring guide.* Canada: Alberta Health Services.

Driscoll, J. (2000) *Practising clinical supervision: a reflective approach.* London: Baillière Tindall.

Engeström, Y. (2001) Expansive learning at work: toward an activity theoretical reconceptualisation. *Journal of Education and Work,* 14(1): 133–156.

Fish, D. (1989) *Appreciating Practice in the Caring Professions: Re-focussing Professional development and practitioner research.* Oxford: Butterworth-Heinemann.

Freeth, D., Hammick, M., Reeves, S., Koppel, I. and Barr, H. (2005) *Effective interprofessional education: Development, delivery and evaluation.* London: Blackwell.

General Medical Council (2009) *Tomorrow's doctors.* London: General Medical Council.

Gibbs, G. (1998) *Learning by doing: a guide to teaching and learning methods.* Oxford: Further Education Unit, Oxford Brookes University.

Goppe, N. (2011) *Mentoring and supervision in health care* (2nd edition). New York: Sage Publications.

Greenhalgh, T. and Hurwitz, B. (1998) *Narrative based medicine: dialogue and discourse in clinical practice.* London: BMJ Books.

Hammick, M., Freeth, D., Koppel, I., Reeves, S. and Barr, H. (2007) A best evidence systematic review of interprofessional education: BEME Guide no. 9. *Medical Teacher* **29**(8): 735–751.

Hayes, E.F. (2005). Approaches to mentoring: how to mentor and be mentored. *Journal of the American Academy of Nurse Practitioners*, **17**, 442–445.

Healthcare Inspectorate Wales (2009) Report of a review in respect of Mr D and the provision of Mental Health Services, following the homicide of Father Paul committed in March 2007. Available from **www.hiw.org.uk.**

Health Professional Council (2009) *Standards for Education and Training*. London: HPC.

Hean, S., and Craddock, D. (2009) Learning theories and interprofessional education: a users guide. *Learning in Health and Social Care*, 8(4): 250–262.

Hean, S., Craddock, D. and Hammick, M. (2012) Theoretical insights into interprofessional education: AMEE Guide No. 62. *Medical Teacher*, **34**(2): e78–101.

Jenson, G.M., Shephard, K.F., Gywer, J. and Hack, L.M. (1999) *Expertise in physical therapy Practice*. USA: Butterworth Heinemann.

Johns, C. (2006) Becoming a reflective practitioner (2nd edition). UK: Wiley-Blackwell Publishing.

Johns, C. (2009) Becoming a reflective practitioner (3rd edition). UK: Wiley-Blackwell Publishing.

Johnson, D.W. and Johnson, R.T. (2009) An educational psychology success story: social interdependence theory and cooperative learning. *Educational Researcher*, 38(5): 365–379.

Lait, J., Suter, E., Arthur, N. and Deutschlander, S. (2011) Interprofessional mentoring: enhancing students' clinical learning. *Nurse Education in Practice*, **11**: 211–215.

Laming, Lord (2009) *The protection of children in England: a progress report*. London: The Stationery Office.

Lave, J. (1988) *Cognition in practice*. Cambridge: Cambridge University Press.

Lave, J. and Wenger, E. (1991) *Situated learning – legitimate peripheral participation*. Cambridge: Cambridge University Press.

Law, S. (2011) Using narratives to trigger reflection. *The Clinical Teacher*, 8: 147–150.

Locke, A. (2008) Developmental coaching: bridge to organizational success. *Creative Nursing*, **14**(3): 102–110.

Marshall, M. and Gordon, F. (2005) Interprofessional mentorship: taking on the challenge. *Journal of Integrated Care*, 13(2): 38–41.

Marshall, M. and Gordon, F. (2010) Exploring the role of the interprofessional mentor. *Journal of Interprofessional Care*, 24(4): 362–374.

Nursing and Midwifery Council (2008a) *The code: standards of conduct, performance and ethics for nurses and midwives*. London: NMC.

Nursing and Midwifery Council (2008b) *Standards to support learning and assessment in practice*. London: NMC.

Nursing and Midwifery Council (2010) *Standards for pre registration nursing education*. London: NMC.

Reeves, S., Goldman, J. and Oandasan, I. (2007) Key factors in planning and implementing interprofessional education in health care settings. *Journal of Allied Health*, **36**(4): 231–235.

Reeves, S., Zwarenstein, M., Goldman, J., Barr, H., Freeth, D., Koppel, I. and Hammick, M. (2010) The effectiveness of interprofessional education: key findings from a new systematic literature review. *Journal of Interprofessional Care*, 24(3): 230–241.

Schon, D. (1983) *The reflective practitioner: how professionals think in action*. New York: Basic Books.

Secretary of State for Health (2001) *Learning from Bristol*. London: The Stationery Office.

Secretary of State for Health (2003) *The Victoria Climbié Inquiry*. London: The Stationery Office.

Sharland, E., Taylor, I., Jones, L., Orr, D. and Whiting, R. (2007) *Interprofessional education for qualifying social work*. Great Britain: Social Care Institute for Excellence.

Sheffield Hallam University (2010) *Interprofessional Capability Framework*. Available from: **http://www. hsaparchive.org.uk/doc/resources/icf2010.pdf/at_ download/file.pdf.** Accessed July 2012.

Shimazoe, J. and Aldrich, H. (2010) Group work can be gratifying: understanding and overcoming resistance to cooperative learning. *College Teaching*, **58**: 52–57.

Torbay Safeguarding Children Board (2010) Serious Case Review. Available from **www.torbay.gov.uk/ c18-execsumm.pdf.**

Vygotsky, L.S. (1978) *Mind in Society. The development of higher psychological processes*. Cambridge, MA: Harvard University Press.

Zwarenstein, M., Atkins, J., Barr, H., Hammick, M., Koppel, I. and Reeves, S. (1999) *A systematic review of interprofessional education*. Journal of Interprofessional Care, **13**(4): 417–424.

Zwarenstein, M., Reeves, S., Barr, H., Hammick, M., Koppel, I. and Atkins, J. (2001) Interprofessional education: effects on professional practice and health care outcomes (Cochrane Review). Available from The Cochrane Library, Oxford.

# CHAPTER 7

# CHALLENGES TO EFFECTIVE INTERPROFESSIONAL WORKING

## LEARNING OBJECTIVES

*By the end of this chapter you should be able to:*

- Identify the challenges to effective interprofessional working

- Critically assess the impact that the identified challenges have on providing effective health and social care delivery

- Suggest ways in which interprofessional working can be enhanced

- Be aware of the differing professional, regulatory and statutory requirements which impact on the interprofessional approach to the exercise of duty of care.

## THE CHALLENGES TO SUCCESSFUL INTERPROFESSIONAL WORKING

In previous chapters, we have considered the essential factors which, if considered as a whole, contribute towards effective interprofessional working.

These factors include:

- UK health and social care policies and legislation
- Teams, teamwork and team dynamics
- Leadership and expertise
- Communicating with each other
- Interprofessional learning

It is now recognized that a single profession or individual can no longer deliver the complex patient care that is demanded in the 21st century. Interprofessional collaboration is essential to the successful achievement of an integrated care system that will enhance patient outcome. Changes in the structure and functioning of the NHS are continuing to take place to facilitate interprofessional collaboration.

Periods of change are, however, uncomfortable and frequently meet with resistance. The transition towards interprofessional working is no exception and it is important to identify the problems, issues and needs that may arise during this period of change. D'Amour and Oandasan (2005) identified three elements that determine how collaboration develops and is consolidated in health care teams:

1 **Systemic factors** – conditions outside the organization
2 **Organizational factors** – conditions within the organization
3 **Interactional factors** – interpersonal relationships between team members

The environment in which interprofessional collaboration takes place is influenced by systemic factors. In a professional practice setting, two of the elements are operating: the organization (organizational factors) and the team (interactional factors). The dynamics of interprofessional collaboration are influenced by all three elements.

In this final chapter, we will use these three elements to explore the potential challenges that exist to successful interprofessional collaboration and explore practical solutions to removing these challenges.

# SYSTEMIC FACTORS

Systemic factors are those factors outside of the organization that impact, either negatively or positively, on interprofessional working. These factors include the professional system and the social system.

## The professional system

The professional system has a significant impact on the development of effective interprofessional working. This is because the professional system appears to run counter to the philosophy of collaboration. In this section, we will consider a number of different aspects of the professional system including:

- professional socialization
- professional language
- professional tribes and territories
- professional codes of conduct
- professions and professionalization.

## Professional socialization

Professional socialization has been defined by Merton *et al.* as:

> ❝ *the process by which people selectively acquire the values and attitudes, the interests, skills and knowledge – in short, the culture – current in groups of which they are, or seek to become a member.*
>
> Merton et al. *(1959, cited in Clouder, 2003, p. 213)*

Early studies of professional socialization describe a process whereby health and social care students are shaped and moulded into 'good' or 'ideal' professionals. This suggests that the student is a passive recipient of knowledge and skills and internalizes the profession's culture completely, without question.

Today, however, a different approach is taken to professional socialization, which is based on 'socialization as interaction' (Ajjawi and Higgs, 2008). This view on professional socialization suggests that a student enters the social world of a profession and, through face-to-face communication with others, establishes what it is to be a professional. The profession has a structure that is created by the way in which members of the profession structure its activities. This structure may, however, be modified over time as new shared understandings are negotiated through the process of professional socialization of newcomers, for example, students. In this approach to professional socialization the student is not passive but is actively using their personal experience to shape their perceptions of their profession.

The process of professional socialization begins as soon as a student enters their professional education programme. The student becomes immersed in the philosophies, values and theoretical perspectives inherent in their profession. Each profession is established on different philosophies, values and theoretical bases. Within an interprofessional team, these differences between the various professionals are potential sources of conflict and as a consequence may hinder the development of effective interprofessional working. Table 7.1 illustrates the values, philosophies and theoretical differences of members of an interprofessional team.

**Table 7.1   The values, philosophies and theoretical differences of members of an interprofessional team**

|  | Doctors | Nurses | Social workers |
|---|---|---|---|
| **Values** | ● Advocate saving life | ● Advocate humanism | ● Advocate quality of life |
| **Questions asked by professionals** | ● Disease oriented e.g. What is the diagnosis? What is the prognosis? What are the symptoms? | ● Patient oriented e.g. What will help this patient to function as well as possible? What support does this patient have at home? | ● Groups or individual clients e.g. What services are available for elderly clients? What social services does this client need? |

*(Continued)*

**Table 7.1  The values, philosophies and theoretical differences of members of an interprofessional team (Continued)**

| | Doctors | Nurses | Social workers |
|---|---|---|---|
| **Treatments and management goals for the patient/client** | ● Based on the medical model. Identifying signs and symptoms. Diagnosing the disease. Treating the disease. Curing the disease | ● Based on the health/illness model. Identifying the patient's health/illness needs. Helping the patient with the activities of daily living. Interested in the holistic view of the patient | ● Based on psycho-social model. Using personality and social resources to improve the situation |
| **Professional expectations** | ● Expert<br>● Full responsibility for care of patient<br>● Leader | ● Supportive, nurturing<br>● Teaching, mentoring<br>● Enabling of self-direction<br>● Makes a difference<br>● Teamwork | ● Trustworthy<br>● Shared responsibility<br>● Active listener<br>● Honest<br>● Reliable |

**Solutions**  A strategy that could be used to overcome this potential source of conflict is for each profession to be explicit about its philosophy and to be prepared to share its values beyond the confines of its professional boundaries. Time should be set aside at team meetings for team members to explore and discuss their different philosophies, values and theoretical bases. Open discussion of differing perspectives can act as a stimulus for new questions and development of the team. This will help the team members to recognize and value the diversity that the different professionals bring to the team. The team will then be able to build on each other's strengths and work together more effectively.

## Differences in professional language

Different professional groups use language very differently. Even when different professions use the same words, the words may mean different things. For example, the term 'service user' may refer to a patient, a client, the family, other service agencies or the community in general. Another example is the term 'assessment'. Assessments are carried out by community nurses, doctors and social workers but the process, context and outcome is very different to each of the professions.

Differences in professional language create a real challenge to the development of collaboration and successful interprofessional working. It means that communication is hindered as the professionals may not be able to understand each other or alternatively they may believe they have understood each other, when actually their interpretations of the conversations are very different as a result of the different meanings that have been attached to specific words.

Unless different professionals are able to effectively communicate with each other and with the patient, family and carers, interprofessional working and hence integrated care will not become a reality.

### Solutions

- **Interprofessional education**
  Interprofessional education provides an opportunity for all health and social care professionals to discover that different professions may use language very differently. Learners will be able to develop an understanding of the language from the perspective of the different professionals. At the same time, the learner will be able to clarify the meaning of words from their own profession.

- **Develop a common language**
  Another strategy is for the team to decide on a common language/common terminology that they are going to use. This will involve identifying terms that mean something different to different professional groups. The team will then need to explore and discuss the terms before agreeing on a common definition for each. A good example would be the one given above, relating to assessment. If they wished to introduce an interprofessional assessment tool, they would first have to come to a common definition for assessment, which was understood by all team members.

## Reflective activity

As a health or social care professional you use jargon and acronyms as part of your everyday language. List the jargon and acronyms that you use as part of your role. For each one consider the following:

- whether a patient would know what it means

- would a colleague from another profession understand what you meant if you said it or wrote it down?

- what strategies could you use to ensure that everyone in your interprofessional team understands what you are saying?

## Professional tribes and territories

Some professionals see interprofessional working as a threat to their professional identity, fearing that traditional boundaries between health and social care professionals will disappear. When we feel under attack, our natural reaction is to retreat into our professional tribe within boundaries and territory with which we are familiar. This may be a natural reaction to conflict and change – resist and defend your tribe at all costs – but it is important that health and social care professionals are able to make this transition and are, thus, able to effectively collaborate within an interprofessional team.

So what is a tribe? As people banded together to constitute primitive societies thousands of years ago, the first major form of organization to emerge was the tribe. The tribe's key function was to infuse a distinct sense of social identity and belonging, thereby strengthening people's ability to bond and survive as individuals and as a collective. A classic tribe may be tied to a specific territory and the exploitation of resources found there. In different tribes, the members speak different languages, practice different rituals and may share some language and rituals with members of other tribes. If we consider this definition of a classic tribe we can see that the notion of 'tribes' and 'tribalism' are useful metaphors when discussing health and social care professions.

Within the definition of a classic tribe, territory is mentioned. A territory refers to an area in which one has rights and responsibilities. Sometimes the area is a concrete space, for example, a ward or department; sometimes it is a sphere of knowledge; and sometimes it refers to elements of both (Dombeck, 1997). Think about how you would introduce yourself at an interprofessional meeting, you might say, for example:

- I am Samantha, I am a social worker working with the elderly in residential care.
- I am Mason, a trainee assistant practitioner on placement in a residential care home.

In these introductions, both Samantha and Mason have described themselves in terms of who they are, their profession, their place of work and their position within an organization. As Samantha and Mason are introducing themselves, they are also staking out their territories and their boundaries. It is therefore not surprising that territorial and tribal issues arise in interprofessional practice, which may impact on the provision of safe, high quality care that patients receive.

### Solutions

- **Articulating professional identity**
  It is important that individual professionals know and are able to articulate their own professional identity before engaging with interprofessional working. It is difficult to work collaboratively if you are unsure of your

own professional identity. Individual professionals must consider what their unique contribution to the interprofessional team is, both as a professional and as a person. For example, what unique knowledge, skills, and professional and personal qualities do you as a nurse, radiographer, midwife, social worker or physiotherapist bring to the interprofessional team and thus to the care and management of patients? If professionals are able to articulate their uniqueness, they will feel less threatened when collaborating with other professionals.

● **Interprofessional working**
It is important that interprofessional working is seen as integrated working and not as a blurring or dismantling of traditional professional boundaries. Integrated working and hence interprofessional working is concerned with different professionals sharing tasks and common skills if there is overlap between the roles of different professional groups, while at the same time each individual retaining their unique combination of skills.

The success of interprofessional working depends on the team identifying clear and distinct boundaries regarding what tasks to share (based upon common skills and tasks), on what occasions, to what effect and where. If the team is able to identify these boundaries then the team will be able to work successfully as an interprofessional team.

Clear boundaries will create trust and respect between the professionals within the team. An appreciation of professional uniqueness and an aware-ness of crossover and overlap in knowledge and skills will also be developed if boundaries are clearly defined.

A team that does not establish clear boundaries around the areas of overlap will lead to ambiguity for the team. Among the team members, there is likely to be role uncertainty, role ambiguity, feelings of inequality, stress and anxiety and a feeling of being unprepared for the role they are expected to carry out. This lack of clarity will hinder successful inter-professional working.

## *Reflective activity*

Identify the unique and distinctive contribution that both you and your profession bring to an interprofessional team. Use the following headings to help guide your thinking:

- knowledge
- skills
- professional qualities
- personal qualities.

## EVIDENCE BASE

Find out more about professional boundaries by reading the following paper:

● Powell, A.R. and Davies, H.T.O. (2012) 'The Struggle to improve Patient Care in the face of Professional Boundaries'. *Social Science & Medicine,* doi:10.1016/j. socscimed.2012.03.049

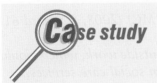

## Case study

### Delivery of effective care involving different health and social care professionals

Mandy is 25-years-old and has a ten-year history of severe bulimia nervosa. Much of her life has revolved around binge eating and vomiting 10–15 times daily and compulsively exercising two hours per day. She spends between £50–£75 per day on food and regularly steals money from her parents and has accumulated a large credit card debt to pay for her food. Mandy describes her life as chaotic, and she is finding it increasingly difficult to hold down her job as shop assistant. Her clothing is baggy and she appears permanently cold and restless. She has admitted suicidal thoughts but has not attempted suicide. She lives at home and is verbally abusive towards her mother, preventing her mother

from caring for her. Her father and sister refuse to acknowledge that she has an eating disorder. No friends visit or come round to the house because Mandy hides plastic bags filled with vomit around the house. Mandy's parents are extremely concerned for their daughter's life.

With reference to the case study:

● List the statutory, voluntary, and community organizations that may be involved with the care of Mandy.

● List the health and social care professionals that are most suited to providing care for Mandy.

● For each health and social care professional listed, identify the unique contribution that they make to the care needs of Mandy.

● Put the professionals on your list in the order that show their importance in:

    – supporting and enabling Mandy to live her life
    – supporting Mandy's parents and sister.

### Professional codes of conduct, performance and ethics

Professional codes of conduct, performance and ethics are frequently cited as potential challenges to interprofessional working. But is this just a myth or is it a reality?

A code of conduct outlines what characteristics professionals should have and how they should act (Banks, 2010). The existence of a code of conduct is often regarded as a prerequisite to acceptance as a profession. This makes the code of conduct an integral part of the professional system. It has been suggested that codes of conduct serve the interests of the profession itself as well as protecting the interests of those whom the profession serves. If this is the case, the codes are promoting professional exclusivity and professional distinctiveness, which may potentially compromise interprofessional working. If we review various codes of conduct we can see that they do contain statements of professional self-interest, for example:

> " *You must behave with honesty and integrity and make sure that your behaviour does not damage the public's confidence in you or your profession.*
>
> Health Professions Council (HPC) (2008, Standard 13)

> " *You must uphold the reputation of your profession at all times.*
>
> Nursing and Midwifery Council (NMC) (2008, Standard 61)

> " *You must not behave in a way, in work or outside work, which would call into question your suitability to work in social care services.*
>
> General Social Care Council (GSCC) (2010, Section 5.8)

However, despite these statements, which clearly demonstrate professional self-interest, the codes do explicitly address cooperation and collaboration between the different health and social care professions, for example:

> " *Working openly and co-operatively with colleagues and treating them with respect.*
>
> GSCC (2010, Section 6.5)

> " *Recognizing and respecting the roles and expertise of workers from other agencies and working in partnership with them.*
>
> GSCC (2010, Section 6.7)

> " *You must work co-operatively within teams and respect the skills, expertise and contributions of your colleagues.*
>
> NMC (2008, Standard 24)

> " *You must be willing to share your skills and experience for the benefit of your colleagues.*
>
> NMC (2008, Standard 25)

> " *You must also communicate appropriately, co-operate, and share your knowledge and expertise with other practitioners, for the benefit of service users.*
>
> HPC (2008, Standard 7)

> " *Respect the skills and contributions of your colleagues.*
> *Communicate effectively with colleagues within and outside the team.*
>
> GMC (2009, p. 22)

Professional codes of conduct are therefore providing a firm foundation for effective interprofessional working. In fact, if the codes are viewed in their totality, they reveal very similar aims, values and guidelines. This suggests that the areas of convergence of opinion far outweigh views that would provide a focus for conflict. So, perhaps it is just a myth that the codes are compromising interprofessional working.

## Professions and professionalization

By definition, belonging to a profession and the process of **professionalization** potentially inhibit the development of collaborative practice.

**professionalization** Is the process by which an occupation elevates itself to the level of a profession

So how is a profession defined? Professions tend to have certain qualities in common:

- Membership of the profession is usually restricted and regulated by a professional association, for example Nursing and Midwifery Council (NMC), Health Professions Council (HPC), General Social Care Council (GSCC), General Medical Council (GMC).
- Professions usually have a great deal of autonomy, setting rules and enforcing discipline themselves.
- Professions are generally exclusive, for example, you cannot practice nursing, radiography, medicine, social work without being registered with a professional body.
- Members of a profession receive an extensive period of education and training prior to practising.
- Professions have an explicit code of conduct for practice.
- Professions have a philosophy of public service and altruism.

If we consider these common qualities of a profession, it can be seen that the concept of a profession is promoting exclusivity, territorial boundaries and distinctiveness. These factors are diametrically opposed to the factors that promote interprofessional working.

Historically, there were only three professions: medicine, law and ministry. Nursing and social work were categorized as semi-professions because of perceived limitations of their knowledge base, training and autonomy (Etzioni, 1969).

As we move towards interprofessional working, it is this hierarchy, created by categorizing the professional groups into professions (higher professions), and semi professions (lower professions), that is having a significant impact on the development of collaborative practice.

Hammick *et al.* (2009) have developed a set of core values that support a culture of being interprofessional. As you will see in Box 7.1 these core values reflect the solutions we have identified through discussing the different aspects of the professional system.

## BOX 7.1

### Core values of being interprofessional

- A caring disposition towards your colleagues

- Respect for everyone in the collaborative team, including the patient and significant others

- Confidence in what you know and what you don't know, and in what others know

- A willingness to engage with others rather than taking a detached view of proceedings

- An approachable attitude and showing a willingness to share what you know as a means to the best possible outcome for the user of your service.

Adapted from: Hammick *et al.* (2009 p. 23)

## The social system

Equality between professionals is one of the basic requirements of collaborative practice. However, within the health and social care professions power differences exist between the different professions. These power differences are most acute between the nursing and medical professions and are based on gender stereotypes and different social status. The boundaries between the nursing and medical professions can be traced back to when these professions emerged. In the 19th century, the medical and nursing professions evolved separately for reasons bound up with the class divisions and gender barriers of Victorian Britain. The result was that, traditionally, males from the higher socio-economic classes have dominated medicine, while females from the middle socio-economic classes have dominated nursing.

Today, the picture is different and the gender mix of these two professions has changed. Since the early 1990s more than half of all new medical students are female and women now form a majority of entrants to most speciality training. By 2017 women doctors will outnumber male doctors in the UK (Khan, 2011). In nursing, there has been a rise in men entering the profession over the last few decades, but it has been small and slow. Fifty years ago there were 1 in 100 male nurses, in 2012 this has risen to one in ten nurses on the NMC register now being male (NMC, 2011). The profession of nursing has also changed substantially, with nurses now taking on new and different roles and responsibilities, for example, the introduction of nurse consultants, nurse specialists and nurse prescribing.

Despite these changes, however, the nurse–doctor relationship still remains problematic. It is apparent that the power imbalance, arising from gender stereotypes, is still preventing effective collaboration between doctors and nurses (Power and Davies, 2012; Mackintosh and Sandall, 2010; Silbey, 2009).

It is crucial that nurses are considered equal partners with doctors if collaborative relationships are to be established.

# ORGANIZATIONAL FACTORS

The organizational setting may help or hinder interprofessional collaboration. In this section, we will consider the organizational factors that are potential challenges to effective collaboration within health and social care settings. These factors include: organizational structure, organizational philosophy, styles of leadership, team resources, methods of communication and professional routines and schedules.

## Organizational structure

Organizational changes have a tendency to reflect changes in the environment that have been triggered by wider social, political and economic changes. As a result, organizations develop at different rates and in doing so create structures, boundaries, finances, timescales and priorities that reflect their role and function.

Historically the NHS has been based on a traditional hierarchical structure. Successful integrated care relies on successful collaboration between health and social care professionals and this can only occur if the traditional hierarchical structure of the NHS is replaced with a more horizontal structure. Progress towards a more horizontal structure has occurred since 1997, with the publication of the White Paper *The New NHS, Modern – Dependable* (Department of Health, 1997) but 15 years later there is still some resistance to these changes by those professions that previously held powerful positions within the hierarchical structure.

Horizontal structures facilitate shared decision-making and open and direct communication, which are important factors in developing teamwork and thus fostering effective interprofessional collaboration.

## Lack of organizational philosophy

It is important that the organization's philosophy supports interprofessional collaboration among health and social care professionals. For example, a philosophy that values trust and respect, participation in planning and decision making, open and direct communication, partnership, innovative working practices, fairness, diversity and interdependence is crucial for the development of effective collaboration within health and social care teams (Carnwell and Carson, 2008).

**interdependence**
Is the occurrence of a reliance on interactions among professionals whereby each is dependent on the other to accomplish their goals and tasks.

## Ineffective leader

Team leaders can make or break a team. When developing an interprofessional team the team leader must specifically be able to:

- convey the vision of collaborative practice to the team members
- motivate the individual team members to engage in collaborative practice
- create an environment within which collaborative practice will flourish.

For a complete list of all the factors that make a team leader effective, you should refer to Chapter 4. In Chapter 4 we also identified that the leadership style most suitable for an interprofessional team leader was a combination of leadership styles, those being transactional and transformational.

If a team leader is ineffective, the team will eventually cease to function as a team. The team members will no longer be committed to the team's shared common goals and objectives and, as a consequence, the delivery of care to patients may become fragmented.

### Solutions: The selection of an appropriate team leader

It is important that a team leader is selected for his or her leadership skills rather than on the basis of status, hierarchy or availability. If this approach is taken to the selection of the team leader, the development of collaboration within an interprofessional team should be assured.

## Lack of team resources

Lack of resources for the team will make it more difficult to develop effective interprofessional working. For example, sufficient time needs to be made available to enable team members to share information, develop interprofessional relationships and address team issues. A lack of available time may lead to the team not developing as effectively as it might. This is because both time and energy are required by all the team members to create a climate in which teamwork will flourish.

Space also needs to be made available. It is important that the team have space in which to meet for both formal and informal occasions. For example, a meeting room with all the appropriate facilities should be available for team meetings, audit meetings and multidisciplinary team (MDT) meetings. Ideally there should also be a shared rest room/coffee room where members of the team can meet informally. If there is a lack of space, it will be difficult for members of the team to communicate face to face. Also, the opportunity for mutual support, trust and respect to develop among the team members will be considerably reduced if there are no spaces available for meeting.

### Solutions

**Regular team meetings** Team meetings should be held on a regular basis to provide an opportunity for the team leaders and members to meet and communicate face to face about matters that affect the team. Commitment to attending a team meeting is higher if the meeting has a regular 'slot' in the calendar. If staff know that the team meeting is held on the first Tuesday of the month between 2.00 p.m. and 3.30 p.m., then team members can schedule their other work commitments around the meeting (see Chapter 5 for further details on team meetings).

**Allocation of dedicated space**   Space is often at a premium within organizations, but it is extremely important that an organization gives consideration to providing space-sharing opportunities to health and social care professionals working in the same team.

## Inadequate communication mechanisms

Lack of standardized documentation, for example, patient records; lack of interprofessional standards, policies and protocols; and lack of formal meetings involving all team members, for instance, team meetings, will inhibit the development of collaboration within interprofessional teams.

### Solutions

**Standardized protocols**   The introduction of standardized communication protocols would enable the transmission of concise, salient information across professional boundaries, overcoming gendered and professional hierarchies (Mackintosh and Sandall, 2010).

## Reflective activity

Think about the interprofessional team in which you are currently working and consider the following points:

- Identify and read your team's/organization's interprofessional standards policies and protocols.

- Identify the documentation that your team use that is unified and standardized for all professionals to use.

- Can you identify any documentation that is not standardized? If you can, develop a standardized document that could be used by all professionals within your team.

## Differences in schedules and professional routines

Different professions differ in the arrangements adopted to accomplish their work and the way in which they work, which can create a barrier to effective interprofessional working. Differences in the length of the working day may prevent members of the interprofessional team attending meetings. For example, GPs plan their time around the needs of patients, and thus hold surgeries in the morning and the afternoon into the evening. GPs, therefore, would not be able to attend meetings during surgery times. As the majority of meetings are held during 'normal' working hours, that is, 9.00 a.m. to 5.00 p.m., this would preclude GPs from attending the majority of meetings.

Different professionals work to different timescales to complete specific tasks. GPs, for example, may work quickly and make a number of assessments and decisions for their patients each day. However, a social worker may undertake long-term casework with a small number of clients. This may also result in interprofessional misunderstanding and conflict.

### Solutions

**Virtual meetings** One possible solution may be to use virtual team meetings. This resource is invaluable as it allows for team members, who are not located on the same sites, to participate in the team meeting without the restrictions on time from travelling.

**Communication board**  A further solution would be to provide a communication board. Staff unable to attend a meeting could post messages for consideration at the meeting.

## INTERACTIONAL FACTORS

Collaboration is a process that occurs between individuals. Therefore, ultimately, it does not matter whether the government or the organizations or the professions want interprofessional working to happen, it is only those individuals involved who can determine whether or not it will happen. Good interpersonal relationships between members of the interprofessional team are, therefore, essential if collaboration is going to occur. Interactional factors that can potentially create challenges for effective interprofessional working are as follows.

## Professional stereotyping

A stereotype is an association and belief about the characteristics and attributes of a group and its members that shape how people think about and respond to the group (Dovidio *et al.*, 2010, p. 8). In stereotyping, information is limited to some highly visible aspect of a person such as age, sex, race, nationality, occupation or physical appearance. This information generates judgements about what any person belonging to that given group is like and that all people belonging to that given group possess the same characteristics (Gross and Kinnison, 2007).

Stereotypes provide us with a mental image of a person that does not correspond to that individual but to what we infer about that individual. Very often our stereotypes are reinforced by the media, for example, by films, books, music, computer games and television. Stereotypes of health and social care professionals may be reinforced by television programmes, such as *Casualty*, *Holby City* or *ER*.

Although stereotyping is often viewed as something that is socially unde-sirable, it is a human process used by everyone and may have both negative and positive outcomes. Stereotypes can lead to very damaging, negative outcomes for both health and social care professionals and their patients, for example, discrimination may lead to an inability to really know your patient/client, which may mean that you cannot provide quality care for them; this could lead to litigation or dissatisfaction with your chosen profes-sion. Alternatively, stereotypes can be seen as a valid mechanism whereby individuals make sense of their interactions with other groups and may be used to positively guide intergroup behaviours (Hean *et al.*, 2006a). It is this positive outcome of stereotyping that health and social care professionals need to capitalize upon.

The existence of interprofessional stereotypes among health and social care professionals has been demonstrated in a number of studies (Bell and Allain, 2011; Ateah *et al.*, 2010; Hean *et al.*, 2006a). These studies have examined the stereotypes held of other professions by health and social care students who are participating in interprofessional education. All three studies used the same questionnaire which required students to rate other professional groups on nine characteristics: academic ability, professional competencies, leadership, being a team player, being an independent worker, confidence, decision making, interpersonal skills and practical skills. Table 7.2 shows the stereotype ratings that the students who participated in these studies gave of professional groups other than their own.

Stereotypes identified in these three studies included:

- Doctors being rated highest on academic ability, professional competence, leadership, being an independent worker, confidence and decision making
- Nurses and social workers being rated highest on being a team player and on their interpersonal skills
- Doctors being rated lowest on being a team player and on their interpersonal skills
- Nurses being rated lowest on academic ability, decision making and on being an independent worker
- Social workers being rated lowest on academic ability, professional competencies and practical skills.

The tensions arising from health and social care professionals holding these stereotypical beliefs could detract from effective health and social care deliv-ery. These stereotypical perceptions that health and social care professionals have of each other will impact negatively on both interprofessional team-work and on the quality of communication. If interprofessional working is to be effective, it is essential that the stereotypical perceptions held by health and social care students are challenged.

## EVIDENCE BASE

Find out more about professional stereotyping by reading the following articles.

- Ateah, C.A., Snow, W., Wener, P., MacDonald, L., Metge, C., Davis, P., Fricke, M., Ludwig, S. and Anderson, J. (2010) Stereotyping as a barrier to collaboration: Does interprofessional education make a difference? *Nurse Education Today,* **30**(2): 208–213.

- Bell, L. and Allain, L. (2011) Exploring professional stereotypes and learning for interprofessional practice: An example from UK qualifying level social work education. *Social Work Education,* **30**(3): 266–280.

- Hean, S., Macleod Clark, J., Adams, K. and Humphries, D. (2006a) Will opposites attract? Similarities and differences in student' perceptions of the stereotype profiles of other heath and social care professional groups. *Journal of Interprofessional Care,* **20**(2): 162–181.

## *Solutions*

**Interprofessional education**    The overarching aim of interprofessional education is to ensure that health and social care students learn with, from and about each other to facilitate collaboration in practice (CAIPE, 2002). Expected outcomes and effects of interprofessional education specifically related to professional stereotyping include:

- Respects individuality, difference and diversity within and between the professions and all with whom they learn and work: utilizing distinctive contribution to learning and practice

- Sustains the identity and expertise of each profession: presenting each profession positively

- Applies equal opportunity within and between the professions and all with whom they learn and work; but setting aside differences in power and status between professions.

*CAIPE (2011)*

Interprofessional education provides a safe environment in which students can explore and discuss with each other their professional biases and gain an appreciation of professional differences. Part of this exploration will involve the student developing a growing awareness of self.

It is important, however, to remember that professional stereotyping can have positive as well as negative outcomes on interprofessional working. The potential positive outcomes relate to intergroup relations. A number of social science theories have been developed to explain intergroup working and are particularly useful for understanding the complexities of interprofessional working and education.

These theories include:

- **Contact theory** – brings different professional groups in contact with each other, under a range of predetermined conditions that promote positive attitudes to grow between professionals (Hean *et al.*, 2012).

- **Realistic contact theory** – predicts that where groups hold divergent objectives they will have hostile and discriminatory intergroup relationships, whereas where groups have common objectives, conciliatory behaviour between groups will emerge (Hind *et al.*, 2003).

- **Social identity theory** – based on the idea that individuals derive their definition of self from their group memberships. Social identity is the identification of self in terms of one's own social group (known as the in-group) rather than of another group (known as the out-group). In the health and social care context, this would mean that individual practitioners would define themselves as not only individuals, that is, 'I' or 'me', but also according to the profession to which they belong, that is, 'we social workers', 'we nurses' (Hind *et al.*, 2003).

When members of the different social groups interact, they make comparisons between the characteristics of their own group (the in-group) and the characteristics of the other social group with whom they are interacting (the out-group). In this way, group members establish their identity of self. This comparison is called intergroup differentiation and can be monitored by considering the stereotypes that individuals hold of their own group and those they hold of the out-group (Hean *et al.*, 2006b).

So, how can we use the social identity theory and positive stereotyping to help inform interprofessional working and interprofessional education? To ensure positive relations between interacting social groups, for example, doctors and nurses, pharmacists and doctors, nurses and radiographers, it is important that when group members are making their intergroup comparisons they are able to see themselves and members of their in-group as distinctive from other groups (the out-groups) on some characteristics. In a study undertaken by Hean *et al.* (2006b), nursing students identified themselves as distinctive on characteristics that included interpersonal skills, team players and practical skills. In the same study, medical students saw their distinctive characteristics as academic ability, leadership, working independently, decision-making and confidence. Social-work students saw themselves as distinct in interpersonal skills, leadership ability and as team players. If group members fail to perceive themselves as distinct, this may lead to an exaggerated favouritism of the in-group and discrimination against the out-group.

Applying this to an interprofessional educational activity, it can be seen that it is important that professional boundaries are maintained. This will ensure that the distinctiveness of each professional group involved in the activity is retained, facilitating harmonious intergroup relations. The outcome of this will be that students should experience good interprofessional relations and will learn that different professions can get on and as a result stereotypical views of each other may become more positive.

If a group's distinctiveness is threatened, this may result in intergroup conflict. This may occur if there is a disagreement between the stereotypes that students hold of their in-group and the stereotypes held of this group by students of other professions. In Hean *et al.*'s (2006b) study, for example, while occupational therapy students believed their group were distinctive on characteristics of inter-personal skills and being team players, this did not match the perceptions of other students. Similarly, radiography students perceived themselves as being distinctive on skills of decision-making and being a team player, but other students did not perceive these strengths. This would suggest that in the examples given, occupational therapy students and radiography students could potentially experience interprofessional conflict during an interprofessional educational activity.

The ability to identify areas of potential interprofessional conflict is important if interprofessional education is to achieve its overall aim of promoting effective interprofessional working. It is, however, equally important to identify situations where other student groups (out-groups) have more positive perceptions of a particular group than its members (in-group). In these circumstances, unrealistic expectations could be placed on each other during an interprofessional activity. Hean *et al.* (2006b) found that other professional groups had positive perceptions of the interpersonal skills of nurses. They suggest that this may lead students from other professions to expect student nurses to be more skilled as communicators and team players than the nurses can demonstrate. This could potentially lead to frustration and anxiety during group activities.

It can be seen that applying the social identity theory to group interactions within an interprofessional context is useful for enhancing our understanding about interprofessional learning processes, the potential positive outcomes of professional stereotyping and the development of effective collaboration in practice.

## Lack of willingness to collaborate

To effectively implement collaborative practice, health and social care professionals must be willing to commit to a collaborative process. There are a number of reasons why individuals may lack a willingness to collaborate, including lack of agreement on the aims of the team or over-ambitious aims; lack of commitment and support from leaders of the team or organization; perceived lack of time for collaboration; lack of shared common goals by team members; lack of clearly stated objectives for the team and lack of group cohesion, due to a lack of professional consistency in the team.

### Solutions

**Effective team building**  Team building will facilitate the development of an effective interprofessional team, whereby health and social care professionals are willing to engage in collaborative practice. It is important, therefore, that team leaders expend both time and energy in building a team. Team building is not a one-off activity but is a continuous process that not only requires commitment from the team leader but also from all the team members.

Factors that will encourage individuals to participate and make a commitment to interprofessional collaboration include:

- shared common goals which are clear and achievable
- open communication between team members and between team members and the team leader
- a supportive transformational team leader
- time to attend interprofessional education courses/study days/conferences
- time for dialogue and discussion, for example, team meetings
- morale support and team spirit
- the roles and responsibilities of team members being clearly articulated and understood by all the team members
- all team members participating fully in the team's activities.

## Lack of trust

Trust is one of the key elements required for the development of collaborative practice. Building trust requires time, effort, patience and previous positive experiences. Two levels of trust can be identified: at one level, trust is about having confidence in your own role and abilities as a professional, while at another level it is about demonstrating trust towards other professionals. At both levels of trust, that trust depends on skills and knowledge, that is, competence and experience of the professional. Within an interprofessional practice environment, professionals place more trust in other professionals considered to be the most experienced and competent.

A lack of trust between members of an interprofessional team will mean that full use of all the knowledge, skills and experience available within the team will not be made. The team will, therefore, not work as effectively as it might and the health and/or social care provided by the team may be compromised as a result.

Lack of trust may also lead to resistance toward the inclusion of team members on patient cases. Each profession may want to handle the case on its own without fully involving the other team members, because of their lack of understanding of what the other professions can offer.

Lack of trust may also result in a team member hesitating to share professional knowledge with the rest of the team. This will alienate and disempower certain team members, which will adversely affect interprofessional working and the delivery of high-quality patient care. Team members' lack of willingness to share professional knowledge may be due, in part, to a desire on the part of the practitioner to defend their own professional identity (see the section on professional tribes on p. 155).

### Solutions

There are a number of strategies which can be used to facilitate the development of trust between different health and social care professions.

**Interprofessional learning**  Interprofessional learning for health and social care practitioners whether at pre-registration or post-registration level, qualificatory or non-qualificatory, in the academic and/or practice setting will enable practitioners to increase their knowledge of the range of skills of others, understand the roles and responsibilities of other health and social care professionals and gain perspectives of other professionals.

**Recognition of the expertise of team members**  This can be achieved by the team leader establishing an environment in which team members respect one another's knowledge and learn to value one another's differences, so that they are able to build on one another's strengths. In an environment that is supportive of diversity, team members will develop trust in each other and as a result work more effectively together.

**Orientation to the role of each profession**  When a new member joins an interprofessional team, as part of their induction programme, they should be provided with an insight into the roles and responsibilities of the different professionals within the team. This could be achieved by the new member of staff spending a specified period of time shadowing each different professional within the team. Such a process will increase the level of trust that the new member develops with their team members, which will facilitate collaborative practice.

## Reflective activity

Think about when you joined a new team and consider the following points.

- What level of trust did you show towards other professionals within the team?
- What level of trust did the other professionals within the team demonstrate towards you?
- When you joined the team, did lack of trust impact on your ability to work effectively within the interprofessional team?
- How did you develop your knowledge and understanding of the roles and responsibilities of the different professionals within the team?

## Lack of communication

Effective communication is an essential precursor for the development of collaboration among health and social care professionals. There are three main reasons why communication is considered crucial to effective interprofessional collaboration:

- Professionals must have the ability to communicate to other professionals how their individual and professional competence and experience contribute to the patient outcomes and to the overall achievement of the team's shared goals and objectives.

- Effective communication will enable constructive negotiations with other professionals. When working collaboratively, it is important that professionals are able to explore the situation and find a solution that is acceptable not only to the professionals involved but that is also consistent with the team's philosophy, shared goals and objectives. The best approach for negotiation within a team is to adopt a win–win approach, that is, one in which both parties feel positive about the situation when the negotiation is concluded. This will help to maintain a positive working relationship afterwards.

- Open and active communication and active listening is crucial for other factors which influence successful collaboration, for example, mutual respect, sharing or mutual trust.

Lack of communication between health and social care professionals can be due to various reasons. Professionals may perceive that they lack the time required to communicate effectively, for example, pressure of the workplace preventing attendance at meetings, or the inability to actively listen to a colleague. Poor negotiation skills may lead to tensions between individual health and social care practitioners and may also affect the dynamics of the team. For example, with an overly aggressive approach you may overpower the other person to give you what you want whether or not that is in the patient's or team's best interest. This would clearly be damaging to subsequent teamwork and effective collaboration. With a too passive approach, you may simply give in to the other person's wishes. This would clearly not be good for the individual professional.

Information overload, incomplete messages or complex lengthy messages all result in poor communication between different health and social care professionals and between health and social care professionals and their patients. This has the potential to lead to errors in the care and treatment patients receive (see Chapter 4).

## Solutions

**Communication skills training for all health and social care professionals**
Since 2002 all pre-registration health and social care students must be able to demonstrate competence in communication with patients, fellow professionals and other health and social care staff (Department of Health, 2000). It is important that communication skills training does not stop once the professional has qualified, but continues throughout their professional life.

**Interprofessional education**   Most universities have adopted an interprofessional learning approach towards the development of communication skills at a pre-registration level. Using a patient-centred approach, students are

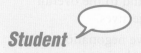

## Student

Behnaz, a second-year adult nursing student, talks about her experiences of completing an interprofessional practice placement within a stroke rehabilitation unit.

"This placement provided me with the opportunity to work closely with a number of different professionals, occupational therapists, physios, and speech and language therapists. Before this placement, I knew very little about what an OT or physio did, but now I have a much better understanding and would feel more confident liaising with them in the future.

The MDT meetings were excellent; you learn such a lot listening to the professionals discussing each patient. It makes you realize how important interprofessional communication is. It is essential if the patient is going to receive high-quality care.

This placement has been so valuable to me, it has helped me to consider the 'wider' picture when caring for patients. I will now feel much happier and more confident to liaise and discuss patients' progress with other professionals and recognize the value of their opinions."

able to learn from and with each other about the advantages and tensions of interprofessional communication in a safe environment.

The introduction of interprofessional practice placements for pre-registration students also enhances communication with and between health and social care professionals, patients and carers.

# RAPID RECAP

Check your progress so far by working through each of the following questions.

1 What are the five factors that contribute to effective interprofessional working?

2 What are the three elements that determine how collaboration develops within health and social care teams?

3 What type of organizational structure needs to be in place if interprofessional working is to be successful?

4 What team resources need to be available if interprofessional working is to be successful?

If you have difficulty with more than one of the questions, read through the section again to refresh your understanding before moving on.

# REFERENCES

Ajjawi, R. and Higgs, J. (2008) Learning to reason: a journey of professional socialisation. *Advances in Health Sciences Education,* **13**(2): 133–150.

Ateah, C.A., Snow, W., Wener, P., MacDonald, L., Metge, C., Davis, P., Fricke, M., Ludwig, S. and Anderson, J. (2010) Stereotyping as a barrier to collaboration: does interprofessional education make a difference? *Nurse Education Today,* **30**(2): 208–213.

Banks, S. (2010) Integrity in professional life: issues of conduct, commitment and capacity. *British Journal of Social Work,* **40**: 2168–2184.

Bell, L. and Allain, L. (2011) Exploring professional stereotypes and learning for interprofessional practice: an example from UK qualifying level social work education. *Social Work Education,* **30**(3): 266–280.

CAIPE (2002) Defining IPE. **www.caipe.org.uk:** Accessed June 2012.

CAIPE (2011) Principles of interprofessional education. **www.caipe.org.uk:** Accessed June 2012.

Carnwell, R. and Carson, A. (2008) The concepts of partnership and collaboration. In *Effective practice in health, social care and criminal justice.* (eds. Carnwell, R. and Buchanan, J.). UK: Open University Press, pp. 3–22. Available from: **http://www.mcgrawhill.co.uk/openup/chapters/9780335229116.pdf.** Accessed June 2012.

Clouder, L. (2003) Becoming professional: exploring the complexities of professional socialization in health and social care. *Learning in Health and Social Care,* **2**(4): 213–222.

D'Amour, D. and Oandasan, I. (2005) Interprofessionality as the field of interprofessional practice and interprofessional education: an emerging concept. *Journal of Interprofessional Care,* **19**(1): 8–20.

Department of Health (1997) *The new NHS, modern – dependable,* London: HMSO.

Department of Health (2000) *A health service of all the talents: developing the NHS workforce.* London: HMSO.

Dombeck, M. (1997) Professional personhood: training, territoriality and tolerance. *Journal of Interprofessional Care,* **11**(1): 9–21.

Dovidio, J.F., Hewstone, M., Glick, P. and Esses, V.M. (2010) *The SAGE handbook of prejudice, stereotyping and discrimination.* Thousands Oaks, CA: Sage.

Etzioni, A. (1969) *The semi-professions and their organization.* New York: Free Press.

Finch, J. (2000) IPE and teamworking – a view from the education providers. *BMJ,* **321**: 1138–1140.

General Medical Council. (2009) *Good medical practice.* London: GMC.

General Social Care Council (2010) *Code of practice for social care workers and employers.* London: GSCC.

Gross, R., and Kinnison, N. (2007) *Psychology for nurses and allied health professionals: applying theory to practice.* London: Hodder Education.

Hammick, M., Freeth, D., Goodsman, D. and Cooperman, J. (2009) *Being interprofessional.* Cambridge: Polity.

Health Professions Council (2008) *Standards of conduct, performance and ethics.* London: HPC.

Hean, S., Craddock, D. and Hammick, M. (2012) Theoretical insights into interprofessional education: AMEE Guide No.62. *Medical Teacher,* **34**(2): e78–101.

Hean, S., Macleod Clark, J., Adams, K. and Humphries, D. (2006a) Will opposites attract? Similarities and differences in student' perceptions of the stereotype profiles of other heath and social care professional groups. *Journal of Interprofessional Care,* **20**(2): 162–181.

Hean, S., Macleod Clark, J., Adams, K., Humphries, D., and Lathlean, J. (2006b) Being seen by others as we see ourselves. The congruence between in-group and out-group perceptions of health and social care students. *Learning in Health and Social Care,* **5**(1): 10–22.

Hind, M., Norman, I., Cooper, S., Gill, E., Hilton, R., Judd, P. and Jones, S.C. (2003) Interprofessional perceptions of health care students. *Journal of Interprofessional Care,* **17**(1): 19–32.

Khan, K. (2011) Medicine – a woman's world. *BMJ,* **19**: d7495.

Mackintosh, N. and Sandall, J. (2010) Overcoming gendered and professional hierarchies in order to facilitate escalation of care in emergency situation: the role of standardized communication protocols. *Social Science and Medicine,* **71**(9): 1683–1686.

Nursing and Midwifery Council (2008) *Code of professional conduct, performance and ethics.* London: NMC.

Nursing and Midwifery Council (2011) Analysis of diversity data: 2011. **www.nmc-uk.org:** Accessed June 2012.

Powell, A.R. and Davies, H.T.O. (2012) The struggle to improve patient care in the face of professional boundaries. *Social Science & Medicine,* doi: 10.1016/j.socscimed. 2012.03.049.

Silbey, S.S. (2009) Taming prometheus: talk about safety and culture. *Annual Review of Sociology,* **35**(1): 341–369.

# APPENDIX

# MAPPING OF CHAPTERS TO NMC STANDARDS AND ESSENTIAL SKILLS CLUSTERS

| Chapter number, title and learning outcomes | NMC Standards for Pre-registration Nursing Education (2010) | | Essential skills cluster | |
| --- | --- | --- | --- | --- |
| | Domain | Competency | Cluster | Skill |
| **1: Introduction – the key concepts of interprofessional working**<br><br>• Identify the key concepts of effective interprofessional working<br><br>• Explain the term 'interprofessional'<br><br>• Be aware of the different organizational levels at which health and social care professionals are required to work together to provide effective delivery of care to the patient and their family and carers. | 1 Professional values | Work in partnership with service users, carers, families, groups, communities and organizations. They must manage risk, and promote health and well-being while aiming to empower choices that promote self-care and safety. | Care, compassion and communication | 4 People can trust a newly qualified graduate nurse to engage with them and their family or carers within their cultural environments in an acceptant and anti-discriminatory manner free from harassment and exploitation. |
| | **2 Communication and interpersonal skills** | 6 Take every opportunity to encourage health-promoting behaviour through education, role modelling and effective communication. | **Organizational aspects of care** | 14 People can trust the newly registered graduate nurse to be an autonomous and confident member of the multidisciplinary or multi-agency team and to inspire confidence in others. |
| | 4 Leadership, management and team working | Work effectively across professional and agency boundaries, actively involving and respecting others' contributions to integrated person-centred care. They must know when and how to communicate with and refer to other professionals and agencies in order to respect the choices of service users and others, promoting shared decision making, to deliver positive outcomes and to coordinate smooth, effective transition within and between services and agencies. | | |

(Continued)

| Chapter number, title and learning outcomes | NMC Standards for Pre-registration Nursing Education (2010) | | Essential skills cluster | |
| --- | --- | --- | --- | --- |
| | Domain | Competency | Cluster | Skill |
| **2: The context of interprofessional working**<br><br>● Identify the relevant UK health and social care policies and legislation that are impacting on interprofessional developments in practice<br><br>● Understand the importance of participating effectively in interprofessional and multi-agency approaches to the delivery of health and social care<br><br>● Be aware of the historical circumstances that initiated the recent interprofessional developments. | 1 Professional values | 4 Work in partnership with service users, carers, families, groups, communities and organizations. They must manage risk, and promote health and well-being while aiming to empower choices that promote self-care and safety. | **Organizational aspects of care** | 11 People can trust the newly registered graduate nurse to safe-guard children and adults from vulnerable situations and support and protect them from harm. |
| | **3: Nursing practice and decision making** | 9 Be able to recognize when a person is at risk and in need of extra support and protection and take reasonable steps to protect them from abuse. | | |
| | 4 Leadership, management and team working | 7 Work effectively across professional and agency boundaries, actively involving and respecting others' contributions to integrated person-centred care. They must know when and how to communicate with and refer to other professionals and agencies in order to respect the choices of service users and others, promoting shared decision making, to deliver positive outcomes and to coordinate smooth, effective transition within and between services and agencies. | | |

| 3: Teams, teamwork and team dynamics | 1 Professional values | | Care, compassion and communication | 1 As partners in the care process, people can trust a newly registered graduate nurse to provide collaborative care based on the highest standards, knowledge and competence. |
|---|---|---|---|---|
| • Describe and define the different types of team<br>• Identify what helps and hinders effective teamwork<br>• Discuss the potential benefits of working in an interprofessional team<br>• Understand the key criteria for evaluating the effectiveness of teams. | | 4 All nurses must work in partnership with service users, carers, families, groups, communities and organizations. They must manage risk, and promote health and well-being while aiming to empower choices that promote self-care and safety. | | |
| | | 6 Understand the roles and responsibilities of other health and social care professionals, and seek to work with them collaboratively for the benefit of all who need care. | Organizational aspects of care | 11 People can trust the newly registered graduate nurse to safeguard children and adults from vulnerable situations and support and protect them from harm. |
| | 2 Communication and interpersonal skills | 8 Respect individual rights to confidentiality and keep information secure and confidential in accordance with the law and relevant ethical and regulatory frameworks, taking account of local protocols. They must also actively share personal information with others when the interests of safety and protection override the need for confidentiality. | | 13 People can trust the newly registered, graduate nurse to promote continuity when their care is to be transferred to another service or person. |

(Continued)

| Chapter number, title and learning outcomes | NMC Standards for Pre-registration Nursing Education (2010) | | Essential skills cluster | |
| --- | --- | --- | --- | --- |
| | Domain | Competency | Cluster | Skill |
| | | | | 14 People can trust the newly registered graduate nurse to be an autonomous and confident member of the multidisciplinary or multi-agency team and to inspire confidence in others. |
| | 3: Nursing practice and decision making | 1 Use up-to-date knowledge and evidence to assess, plan, deliver and evaluate care, communicate findings, influence change and promote health and best practice. They must make person-centred, evidence-based judgments and decisions, in partnership with others involved in the care process, to ensure high quality care. They must be able to recognize when the complexity of clinical decisions requires specialist knowledge and expertise, and consult or refer accordingly. | | |
| | 4 Leadership, management and team working | 6 Work independently as well as in teams. They must be able to take the lead in coordinating, delegating and supervising care safely, managing risk and remaining accountable for the care given. | | |

| 4: Leadership and expertise | 4 Leadership, management and team working | | Organizational aspects of care | |
|---|---|---|---|---|
| • Identify the key elements which relate to effective leadership<br>• Understand the complex nature of expertise<br>• Discuss the relationship between knowledge and expertise<br>• Have insight into how expertise influences the leadership within an interprofessional team. | | 7 Work effectively across professional and agency boundaries, actively involving and respecting others' contributions to integrated person-centred care. They must know when and how to communicate with and refer to other professionals and agencies in order to respect the choices of service users and others, promoting shared decision making, to deliver positive outcomes and to coordinate smooth, effective transition within and between services and agencies. | | 15 People can trust the newly registered graduate nurse to safely delegate to others and to respond appropriately when a task is delegated to them. |
| | | 1 Act as change agents and provide leadership through quality improvement and service development to enhance people's well-being and experiences of health care. | | |
| | | 6 Work independently as well as in teams. They must be able to take the lead in coordinating, delegating and supervising care safely, managing risk and remaining accountable for the care given. | | 16 People can trust the newly registered graduate nurse to safely lead, coordinate and manage care. |

(Continued)

| Chapter number, title and learning outcomes | NMC Standards for Pre-registration Nursing Education (2010) | | Essential skills cluster | |
|---|---|---|---|---|
| | Domain | Competency | Cluster | Skill |
| **5: Communicating with each other**<br><br>• Discuss the fundamental communication skills needed to facilitate effective relationships with patients, carers and health care professionals<br><br>• Identify the methods of communication that enhance effective interprofessional working<br><br>• Discuss the barriers to effective communication. | 1 Professional values | 4 Work in partnership with service users, carers, families, groups, communities and organizations. They must manage risk, and promote health and well-being while aiming to empower choices that promote self-care and safety. | Care, compassion and communication | 6 People can trust the newly registered graduate nurse to engage therapeutically and actively listen to their needs and concerns, responding using skills that are helpful, providing information that is clear, accurate, meaningful and free from jargon. |
| | | 6 Understand the roles and responsibilities of other health and social care professionals, and seek to work with them collaboratively for the benefit of all who need care. | Organizational aspects of care | 11 People can trust the newly registered graduate nurse to safeguard children and adults from vulnerable situations and support and protect them from harm. |
| | 2 Communication and interpersonal skills | 2 Use a range of communication skills and technologies to support person-centred care and enhance quality and safety. They must ensure people receive all the information they need in a language and manner that allows them to make informed choices and share decision making. They must recognize when language interpretation or other communication support is needed and know how to obtain it. | | 13 People can trust the newly registered, graduate nurse to promote continuity when their care is to be transferred to another service or person. |

3 Use the full range of communication methods, including verbal, non-verbal and written, to acquire, interpret and record their knowledge and understanding of people's needs. They must be aware of their own values and beliefs and the impact this may have on their communication with others. They must take account of the many different ways in which people communicate and how these may be influenced by ill health, disability and other factors, and be able to recognize and respond effectively when a person finds it hard to communicate.

4 Recognize when people are anxious or in distress and respond effectively, using therapeutic principles, to promote their well-being, manage personal safety and resolve conflict. They must use effective communication strategies and negotiation techniques to achieve best outcomes, respecting the dignity and human rights of all concerned. They must know when to consult a third party and how to make referrals for advocacy, mediation or arbitration.

5 Use therapeutic principles to engage, maintain and, where appropriate, disengage from professional caring relationships, and must always respect professional boundaries.

(Continued)

| Chapter number, title and learning outcomes | NMC Standards for Pre-registration Nursing Education (2010) | | Essential skills cluster | |
| --- | --- | --- | --- | --- |
| | Domain | Competency | Cluster | Skill |
| | | 7 Maintain accurate, clear and complete records, including the use of electronic formats, using appropriate and plain language. | | |
| | | 8 Respect individual rights to confidentiality and keep information secure and confidential in accordance with the law and relevant ethical and regulatory frameworks, taking account of local protocols. They must also actively share personal information with others when the interests of safety and protection override the need for confidentiality. | | |
| | 4: Leadership, management and team working | 7 Work effectively across professional and agency boundaries, actively involving and respecting others' contributions to integrated person-centred care. They must know when and how to communicate with and refer to other professionals and agencies in order to respect the choices of service users and others, promoting shared decision making, to deliver positive outcomes and to coordinate smooth, effective transition within and between services and agencies. | | |
| 6: Interprofessional learning within a practice environment<br><br>● Discuss the developments in interprofessional learning<br>● Understand situated learning theory | 1 Professional values | 4 Work in partnership with service users, carers, families, groups, communities and organizations. They must manage risk, and promote health and well-being while aiming to empower choices that promote self-care and safety. | Organizational aspects of care | 12 People can trust the newly registered graduate nurse to respond to their feedback and a wide range of other sources to learn, develop and improve services. |

- Create a learning environment within which effective interprofessional learning can take place
- Critically appraise the concept of interprofessional mentorship.

7 Be responsible and accountable for keeping their knowledge and skills up to date through continuing professional development. They must aim to improve their performance and enhance the safety and quality of care through evaluation, supervision and appraisal.

9 Appreciate the value of evidence in practice, be able to understand and appraise research, apply relevant theory and research findings to their work, and identify areas for further investigation.

**2 Communication and interpersonal skills**

6 Take every opportunity to encourage health-promoting behaviour through education, role modelling and effective communication.

**4 Leadership, management and team working**

5 Facilitate nursing students and others to develop their competence, using a range of professional and personal development skills

14 People can trust the newly registered graduate nurse to be an autonomous and confident member of the multidisciplinary or multi-agency team and to inspire confidence in others.

*(Continued)*

| Chapter number, title and learning outcomes | NMC Standards for Pre-registration Nursing Education (2010) | | | Essential skills cluster | |
| --- | --- | --- | --- | --- | --- |
| | Domain | Competency | Cluster | Skill | |
| **7: Challenges to effective interprofessional working**

• Identify the challenges to effective interprofessional working

• Critically assess the impact that the identified challenges have on providing effective health and social care delivery

• Suggest ways in which interprofessional working can be enhanced

• Be aware of the differing professional, regulatory and statutory requirements which impact on the interprofessional approach to the exercise of duty of care. | 1 Professional values | 8 Practise independently, recognizing the limits of their competence and knowledge. They must reflect on these limits and seek advice from, or refer to, other professionals where necessary. | **Organizational aspects of care** | 11 People can trust the newly registered graduate nurse to safeguard children and adults from vulnerable situations and support and protect them from harm. | |
| | 4: Leadership, management and team working | 7 Work effectively across professional and agency boundaries, actively involving and respecting others' contributions to integrated person-centred care. They must know when and how to communicate with and refer to other professionals and agencies in order to respect the choices of service users and others, promoting shared decision making, to deliver positive outcomes and to coordinate smooth, effective transition within and between services and agencies. | | | |

# APPENDIX
# RAPID RECAP ANSWERS

## CHAPTER 1

1 **What are the three mechanisms that need to be in place if interprofessional working is to be successful?**

The three mechanisms which need to be in place if interprofessional working is to be successful are:

- Institutional supports, for example, clear governance models, structured protocols and shared operating procedures
- A good working culture is required through structured information systems and processes, effective communication strategies, conflict resolution policies and regular dialogue between health and social care professionals.
- Environment. Space designs, facilities and the built environment can impact significantly on the effectiveness of interprofessional working.

2 **What is the difference between interprofessional working and multiprofessional working?**

The difference between interprofessional working and multiprofessional working is that with interprofessional working, professionals work together for the mutual benefit of all the professional groups involved. With multiprofessional working, professionals work or learn side by side for a specific task with little collaboration.

3 **What is interprofessional education?**

Interprofessional education is when two or more professions learn from and about each other to improve collaboration and the quality of care.

4 **What is interagency working?**

Interagency working denotes the reciprocal relationship both between and amongst an organization providing a particular service.

## CHAPTER 2

1 **What are the five drivers for interprofessional working?**

The drivers for interprofessional working are:

- The voice of the patient
- Policies and initiatives
- Poor collaborative practice
- Professional developments
- Technological developments.

2 **What three factors are still inhibiting successful interprofessional working?**

The three factors that are inhibiting successful interprofessional working are:

- Lack of collaboration between agencies
- Lack of effective communication
- Lack of adequate training.

3 **What was the purpose of developing Sure Start?**

The aim of Sure Start was to tackle child poverty and social exclusion through integration and co-ordination of services in early education, childcare, and health, employment and family support for pre-school children and their families.

4 **What are the main Department of Health policies that have impacted on the delivery of stroke services in the UK?**

The main Department of Health policies that have impacted on the delivery of stroke services in the UK are:

- *The National Service Framework (NSF) for Older People* (Department of Health, 2001)
- *The National Stroke Strategy* (Department of Health, 2007).
- *Stroke-specific Education Framework* (Department of Health, 2009).

## CHAPTER 3

1 **What are the essential features of a team?**

The essential features of a team are a group of people who:

- Share a common purpose and common goals
- Have a clear understanding of each other's roles and abilities
- Are task oriented and have different but complementary skills
- Have a shared knowledge, skills and resource base and collective responsibility for the outcome of their decisions.

2 **What are the essential characteristics of teamwork?**

The essential characteristics of teamwork are:

- Having a common purpose and common objectives
- Delegation and empowerment
- Different professional contributions
- Having systems in place to facilitate effective communication
- Coordination, cooperation and joint thinking
- Focusing on the patient to provide the best means of serving the patient's interests
- Allowing team members to carry out the team's work and to manage itself as an independent group of people.

3 **What are the five stages of team development?**

The five stages of team development are:

- Forming
- Storming
- Norming
- Performing
- Adjourning.

4 **List Belbin's nine team roles, which he considered were necessary if a team was to be successful.**

Belbin's nine team roles which he considered were necessary if a team was to be successful are:

- Implementer
- Shaper
- Plant
- Resource-investigator
- Monitor evaluator
- Team worker
- Completer-finishers
- Coordinator
- Specialist

5 **What factors contribute towards effective interprofessional teamwork?**

The factors that contribute towards effective interprofessional teamwork are:

- Clear team goal
- Open communication
- Support for innovation

- High levels of participation
- Clear roles and responsibilities
- Competent team members
- Effective time management
- Values diversity
- High level of commitment
- Joint education and training
- Effective conflict resolution
- Moral support and team spirit.

# CHAPTER 4

1 **What are the main types of leadership style?**

The main types of leadership style are:

- Participative leadership
- Situational leadership
- Transactional leadership
- Transformational leadership
- Charismatic leadership
- Authentic leadership.

2 **What leadership styles are usually adopted by an interprofessional team leader?**

The leadership styles that are usually adopted by an interprofessional team leader are transformational leadership and transactional leadership.

3 **What skills and qualities does an effective team leader possess?**

Effective team leaders possess the following skills and qualities:

- honesty, integrity, humility, courage, commitment, confidence, passion, determination and sensitivity
- support the developmental needs of their individual team members
- the ability to balance the demands of the day-to-day tasks and team dynamics so that the needs of everyone involved in completing the task are taken into account
- have a vision and are able to motivate and inspire people to put the vision into practice
- have a high level of self-awareness and know their own strengths and limitations
- the ability to assess the competence levels of their team members and their commitment to completing tasks to achieve the required outcomes.

**4  What are the strands of professional knowledge?**

The strands of professional knowledge are:

- Propositional knowledge
- Personal knowledge
- Non-propositional knowledge
- Social knowledge.

**5  List five of the key characteristics of an expert.**

The key characteristics of an expert are:

- Experts are knowledgeable and have a deep level of propositional knowledge and a large volume of non-propositional knowledge
- Experts are reflective practitioners
- Experts are highly motivated and internally driven
- Experts excel mainly in their own domain
- Experts are faster at performing the skills of their domain
- Experts are fast at solving problems and make few errors
- Experts value the participation of relevant others in the decision-making process
- Experts are patient centred
- Experts share their expertise to help develop expertise in others.

# CHAPTER 5

**1  What are the main methods of verbal communication?**

The main methods of verbal communication are spoken language and non-verbal actions. These may be in the form of formal and informal communication and direct (face-to-face) verbal communication strategies. Formal strategies include team meetings, ward rounds and multi-disciplinary team meetings. Informal communication strategies are more opportunistic and spontaneous.

**2  What are the benefits of multidisciplinary team meetings?**

The benefits of multidisciplinary team meetings are:

- Each different professional contributes independently to the diagnostic treatment or care decisions for a patient case
- They comprise of professionals working across different sector boundaries
- They ensure that all professionals involved get an equal opportunity to listen and to talk about the patients within their care

- They ensure that the patient will receive the most suitable care from diagnosis through treatment to follow-up care and support with the least delay. This will contribute to improved patient outcome.

3 **How do electronic health records and electronic social care records enhance interprofessional communication?**

Electronic records enhance interprofessional communication because they are easier to read, less bulky and reduce the need for professionals to re-record information that has already been recorded by another professional. Currently, different professions use different documentation systems. This results in a variation in the detail of information that is recorded, potentially leading to less than optimal patient care. By standardizing the structure and type of information collected to one central source, any duplication of information/treatment will be avoided and the interprofessional team will be able to work together more effectively.

4 **What factors inhibit interprofessional communication?**

The factors that inhibit interprofessional communication are:

- Inappropriate channel of communication selected, for example, selecting a written method when face-to-face communication would have been better or vice versa
- Distractions, for example other people talking, equipment, noise, televisions, radios, interruptions
- Hierarchy – the hierarchical nature of health care creates power gaps that contribute to less than optimal communication between different professionals and with patients
- Lack of time – to communicate effectively takes time and the pressures of the workplace may result in the health care professionals doing another task or thinking about what they are going to do next at the same time as a message is being communicated to them. As a consequence, the health care professional is not fully concentrating and focusing on the person speaking and this may result in vital information being lost or misinterpreted
- Complex messages – these will increase the chances of the message being misunderstood or misinterpreted
- Ideological differences between health care professions
- Too much information – this may result in information overload
- Different professional language
- Different professional jargon
- Too much communication – may be via the telephone or e-mail or during a ward round or team meeting, with so many communications it can be difficult if not impossible to determine which communications are most critical.

# CHAPTER 6

**1 What are the key features of a community of practice?**

The key features of a community of practice are:

- Communities of practice are everywhere – at home, at work, at university – we all belong to a number of them
- Communities of practice are informally bound by what they do together and by what they have learned through their mutual engagement in these activities
- They develop around things that matter to people
- The practices of a community reflect the members' own understanding of what is important
- Communities of practice are defined by what the community is about; how it functions and what capability it has produced.

**2 List the key points of situated learning theory.**

The key points of situated learning theory are:

- Situated learning recognizes that knowledge is embedded within the context in which it is used and cannot be separated from the activity, context and culture of that situation
- Learners engage in situated learning by negotiating meaning with one another through the use of tools and artefacts such as language, books, music and art
- Learning takes place as a result of participating in 'real' activities that nurture and guide the learner's ability to think
- Learners develop a shared understanding about the purpose of the community and develop a sense of belonging.

**3 What are the key features of a situated-learning environment?**

The key features of a situated-learning environment are:

- It fosters the development of lifelong learning skills
- Situated learning and teaching strategies include critical appreciation; cooperative learning; collaboration; reflection; coaching and narrative
- Learning takes place in the zone of proximal development through interactions between a newcomer and an old-timer
- Learner and facilitator are actively involved in and jointly manage the responsibility for learning
- Situated learning techniques take more time and effort for both the learner and facilitator.

**4 What is the role of an interprofessional mentor?**

The primary role of an interprofessional mentor would be the same as those of a uniprofessional mentor, that is, the facilitation of learning, supervision and assessment of learners in the practice environment. The application of these roles, however, would be related to the learner's interprofessional learning outcomes.

## CHAPTER 7

**1 What are the five factors that contribute to effective interprofessional working?**

The five factors that contribute to effective interprofessional working are:

- UK health and social care policies and legislation
- Teams, teamwork and team dynamics
- Leadership and expertise
- Communicating with each other
- Interprofessional learning.

**2 What are the three elements that determine how collaboration develops within health and social care teams?**

The three elements which determine how collaboration develops within health and social care teams are:

- Systemic factors – conditions outside the organization
- Organizational factors – conditions within organization
- Interactional factors – interpersonal relationships between team members.

**3 What type of organizational structure needs to be in place if interprofessional working is to be successful?**

The type of organizational structure that needs to be in place if interprofessional working is to be successful is a horizontal structure. A horizontal structure, rather than the traditional hierarchical structure, needs to be in place if there is to be successful integrated collaboration between health and social care professionals.

**4 What team resources need to be available if interprofessional working is to be successful?**

The team resources that need to be available if interprofessional working is to be successful are:

- Regular team meetings to provide an opportunity for the team leaders and team members to meet and communicate face to face about matters that affect the team
- Allocation of dedicated space.

# INDEX